**Developments in
Steroid Histochemistry**

Developments in Steroid Histochemistry

A. H. BAILLIE and **M. M. FERGUSON**
Department of Anatomy, The University, Glasgow, Scotland

and

D. McK. HART
Department of Obstetrics, Queen Mother's Hospital, Glasgow, Scotland

1966

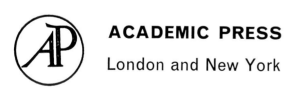

ACADEMIC PRESS
London and New York

ACADEMIC PRESS INC. (LONDON) LTD
BERKELEY SQUARE HOUSE
BERKELEY SQUARE
LONDON, W.1

U.S. Edition published by
ACADEMIC PRESS INC.
111 FIFTH AVENUE
NEW YORK, NEW YORK 10003

Library of Congress Catalog Card Number: 66-30075

Printed in Great Britain by
Robert MacLehose and Company Limited
The University Press, Glasgow

Preface

In recent years, techniques have been evolved that permit the localization in tissue sections of a group of enzymes concerned in steroid metabolism, the hydroxysteroid dehydrogenases. To facilitate evaluation of these histochemical techniques and interpretation of the findings of the numerous investigators in this field, this up-to-date review of the steroid histochemical literature has been prepared, with a discussion of the significance of the results. From a biological standpoint, the work described has serious implications for workers in the fields of renal, hepatic, adrenal and reproductive physiology, and the results are of special consequence in the clinical aspects of endocrine diseases. It is hoped that this account will not only serve as a basis for further histochemical work but will also present the correct image of the subject to the biochemist.

We deeply regret the untimely death of our colleague, and co-author, Dr. A. H. Baillie, before the completion of this book. Dr. Baillie was a dedicated steroid histochemist whose training as an anatomist allowed him to approach the problems of steroid metabolism in terms of cells and tissues.

While we must bear the responsibility for many of the views expressed in this book we should like to acknowledge the encouragement and assistance of several people in preparing this work. Among these we are particularly indebted to Professor G. M. Wyburn, Professor of Anatomy in the University of Glasgow, for research facilities, and the clinicians for providing human tissues. Our sincere thanks are also due to Boots Pure Drug Co. Ltd., Organon Laboratories Ltd., Searle Ltd. and Schering A.G. Berlin for their generous gifts of steroids.

The authors thank the publishers of *Histochemie, Journal of Clinical Endocrinology and Metabolism* and *Journal of Endocrinology* for permission to use in this volume several photographs from their previous papers appearing in these journals.

Finally, we wish to express our gratitude to Academic Press for helpful cooperation in preparing the text.

University of Glasgow
September 1966

M. M. FERGUSON
D. McK. HART

v

Contents

CHAPTER 6

CHAPTER 7

CHAPTER 8

CHAPTER 9

CHAPTER 10

CHAPTER 11

CHAPTER 1

General Considerations

I. INTRODUCTION

The existence in mammalian tissues of a Δ^5-3β-hydroxysteroid dehydrogenase was first established biochemically by Samuels *et al.* (1951), and Wattenberg (1958) coupled this oxidation to the reduction of a tetrazolium salt, making histological localization of the reaction (Fig. 1) possible in tissue sections.

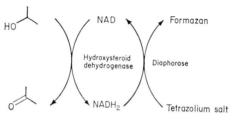

FIG. 1. Mechanism of histochemical demonstration of hydroxysteroid dehydrogenase activity in tissue sections.

Oxidation and reduction reactions are important in steroid, as in other metabolic, pathways, and the literature concerning the biochemical aspects of animal and microbiological steroid dehydrogenations has been reviewed by Talalay (1957, 1965), Talalay and Williams-Ashman (1960). In some instances the enzymes responsible for catalysing the reaction have been extensively purified and kinetic data have been established. This is particularly true of oestradiol-17β-hydroxysteroid dehydrogenase, which, since the original suggestion, in 1952, of transhydrogenase function (Fig. 8) (Hagerman and Villee, 1952, 1953), has been extensively studied and of which a number of parameters of enzyme activity has been documented. In contrast, the existence of other enzymes such as 6β-hydroxysteroid dehydrogenase has only been inferred from the isolation of 6-oxo derivatives, or by the use of crude extracts to demonstrate the reaction (Breuer *et al.*, 1958).

In a similar manner, when the physiological significance of the individual hydroxysteroid dehydrogenases is considered, some, such as the Δ^5-3β-hydroxysteroid dehydrogenase, have a well recognized position in an established biochemical pathway, and accordingly demonstration of this enzyme in a particular tissue is of known significance. On the other hand, certain enzymes with, as yet, poorly defined biochemical roles, present a problem in interpretation when the enzymes are localized in a particular tissue.

1

This review is concerned with the histochemical localization of hydroxy-steroid dehydrogenases, and this limitation immediately introduces advantages and disadvantages. The most important advantage, and indeed the purpose of histochemical work, is the accurate localization of the site of the enzyme reaction. This statement presupposes that the enzyme is in fact being demonstrated at its site of action and where relevant other factors such as enzyme solubility and diaphorase localization must be considered. A further major advantage is the simplicity and speed with which histochemical assays can usually be carried out. One of the disadvantages is that with the hydrogen acceptor, which is the most suitable for histochemical localization, the reaction product cannot be extracted and measured. Further, the end products of the reaction are not isolated, and so the reaction is in fact inferred. Both of these disadvantages may be overcome by simultaneously using standard biochemical techniques, and perhaps, in the future, microchemical methods will allow localization, isolation and quantitation.

Since the original use of a hydrogen acceptor to follow the course of hydroxysteroid dehydrogenations by Wattenberg in 1958, a great deal of histochemical work has been done, but as yet no histochemical review of the literature or of the present status of the subject has appeared. Development has been along two principal pathways. Firstly, there has been a search for new enzymes detectable by a modified Wattenberg technique; secondly, the localization of these enzymes in different species, organs and tissues at different physiological periods and during the development of the organism has been studied. This second aspect, that of tissue and organ localization, will be considered in detail in the rest of the review. The first aspect, a short history of the technical demonstration of the hydroxysteroid dehydrogenases, can conveniently be considered at this point.

Wattenberg (1958) first described the histochemical distribution of Δ^5-3β-hydroxysteroid dehydrogenase in a number of tissues, and Levy et al. (1959a) confirmed the method shortly afterwards. Pearson and Grose (1959a, b) demonstrated 3α- and 17β-hydroxysteroid dehydrogenases, and since then methods for other enzymes have been described; Balogh (1964) visualized 20α-hydroxysteroid dehydrogenase, and techniques for 6β-, 11β-, 12α-, 16α-, 16β- and 20β- hydroxysteroid dehydrogenases have been published (Baillie et al., 1965a, b; 1966a). The remainder of this chapter deals with techniques, specificity and general biochemical considerations.

II. PRE-INCUBATION TECHNIQUES

Steroid-producing organs and target organs for steroid hormones show remarkable species (Wattenberg, 1958; Rubin et al., 1963a) and individual variability (Baillie and Mack, 1966) in activity. Moreover, activity is influenced by the age (Rubin et al., 1963b; Hart et al., 1966) and the sex of the animal (Rubin and Strecker, 1961; Baillie et al., 1966b), by cyclical phenomena (Ikonen et al., 1961; Deane et al., 1962) and by general health and diet (Marx et al., 1963; Kormano et al., 1964). Thus the selection of an animal for histochemical localization of hydroxysteroid dehydrogenases should take account of all these factors. A stress-free environment is of particular importance when the adrenal cortex or gonads are being studied.

Methods of killing the animal before removing the tissue for study are important since they may affect the activity of the enzymes. In all cases there is some degree of stress involved, and this may lead to changes in enzyme activity. In general, the more rapid the method, the less stress involved. Chemical methods using anaesthetics are usually slower than the physical methods such as cervical dislocation, decapitation or cranial trauma. They have the further disadvantage that the agents used are generally lipid-soluble and so may be selectively taken up by steroid-producing tissues, many of which are rich in lipid, and the effects on steroid metabolism of such anaesthetics are not known.

The tissue to be examined should be removed with great care to prevent any compression with forceps; Chayen et al., (1965) state that relatively gentle mechanical pressure can cause a marked increase in mitochondrial glutamic dehydrogenase activity. The time of removal of the tissue after death is also important, since post mortem autolysis and enzyme diffusion may alter the enzyme localization and activity.

The question of fixation of tissues or tissue sections is a controversial one. If the enzyme under investigation is at all soluble then the desirability of fixation or of restricting diffusion is obvious, since, theoretically, only by doing this will accurate localization be possible. Fixation, on the other hand, introduces undesirable factors, such as denaturation of the enzymes and other proteins, so that the system becomes progressively further removed from the physiological norm. The ideal fixative would be a substance which would rapidly diffuse through the tissue causing the proteins only to become more stable and give a minimum of denaturation. Since these parameters are at present difficult to measure, fixation will for the time being be subject to criticism. Whether some loss of activity, and it should be remembered that this would probably be a differential loss, could be accepted for a possible increase in accuracy of localization is a vexed question.

Experiments in this laboratory using a variety of fixatives have indicated that hydroxysteroid dehydrogenases are particularly sensitive to a wide range of reagents, and this was Fuhrmann's (1961) experience with 3β-hydroxysteroid dehydrogenase. Brief formalin vapour fixation of freeze-dried tissues does not seriously impair strongly active hydroxysteroid dehydrogenase and diaphorase activity. For light microscopy, hydroxysteroid dehydrogenase activity is completely abolished by fixation in mercuric chloride, osmium tetroxide and potassium permanganate.

A. SECTIONING

For reasons outlined above dehydrated and wax-embedded tissues are useless for the demonstration of hydroxysteroid dehydrogenases, and unfixed frozen sections only are used. Various techniques exist for rapid freezing of tissues but all carry the risk of ice crystal artifact. Small blocks of tissue permit of rapid and complete freezing, whereas larger portions over 1 cm³ may appear normal round the periphery but contain extensive ice crystal artifact in the centre. As rapid a rate of cooling as possible is desirable and can be obtained by using a freezing substance with a high thermal conductivity. Quenching in liquid nitrogen or on solid carbon dioxide are widely used at present and these methods seem to be satisfactory. Alternatively, the tissue can be placed unfrozen on a chuck which is then immersed in liquid nitrogen. Immersing the tissue to be frozen into a liquid cooled either with liquid nitrogen or solid CO_2 has many theoretical advantages (Fig. 2), but the

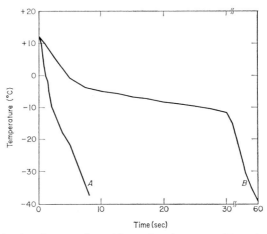

Fig. 2. Graph showing tissue cooling with two freezing agents. Trace A represents muscle cooled in hexane at $-70°$ C, Trace B muscle cooled in a dry tube at $-70°$ C. By courtesy of Dr. J. Chayen.

available liquids are also lipid-solvents and this point will be returned to below. Scott (1933) introduced ethanol and Hoerr (1936) used cooled isopentane, but both of these are viscous at the low temperatures used. Various other mixtures have been tried, and Bell (1952) suggested the use of dichlorofluoromethane (Arcton-6, I.C.I.) for freezing tissues. More recently Bitensky *et al.* (1965) have found that hexane cooled with solid carbon dioxide has proved satisfactory, producing minimal ice crystal artifact.

Tissues can be stored wrapped in Parafilm at $-40°$ C, but Bitensky *et al.* (1965) have pointed out that ice equilibrium occurs at $-40°$ C and do not recommend storage at this temperature for more than a few days. Tissue blocks can be stored at $-70°$ C if it is required to retain them over a longer period.

Sections are cut in a cryostat and although the literature contains numerous references to methods of freezing tissues without causing ice crystal artifact, it is not generally appreciated that the tissue section thaws and refreezes on cutting and is thawed a second time on attaching to the warm cover slip. From this it would appear that the crucial period for ice crystal artifact formation is during the initial freezing of the whole block.

The practice of pre-incubation washing of tissue sections in acetone is widespread, supposedly to give more accurate enzyme localization by removal of lipids (Wattenberg, 1958; Levy *et al.*, 1959a). The overall histochemical technique, however, is satisfactory for localization at a cellular level only of hydroxysteroid dehydrogenase activity (see page 9). In addition Dawson *et al.* (1961) state that Nitro BT formazan is not lipid-soluble, and Levy *et al.* (1959b) found that a pre-incubation wash in acetone abolished Δ^5–3β-hydroxy-steroid dehydrogenase activity in the theca interna of rat ovaries. We have found no advantages in washing tissues in acetone and in fact note a general overall reduction in hydroxysteroid dehydrogenase activity. In some circumstances a short pre-incubation wash in cold buffer may be necessary, if control difficulties are encountered, in the hope of removing some soluble intrinsic substrates. In our opinion pre-incubation washing of any sort should be avoided unless absolutely necessary.

III. INCUBATION TECHNIQUES

It has already been mentioned that the great virtue of the histochemical method for hydroxysteroid dehydrogenase is its simplicity and rapidity. However, there are a number of practical problems to which attention should be paid when establishing the optimum conditions for a particular system. Further, the fact that the technique is a simple one does not exempt it from the dangers of interpretation and assessmen t which are characteristic of more complex methods. A number of the features of the histochemical system raise peculiar difficulties and must be considered in detail.

A. CHOICE OF STEROID SUBSTRATE

This is one of the most important points in the histochemical demonstration of hydroxysteroid dehydrogenases and two features have to be considered. The class of steroid substrate, whether it is a C_{21}, C_{19} or C_{18} steroid, is of great importance, and the labelling of an enzyme '3β-hydroxysteroid dehydrogenase' without defining the substrate used can cause considerable confusion. The second factor requiring consideration concerns the available hydrogen on the steroid used as substrate. Thus steroids with several hydroxyl groups are of use in histochemical work when suitable controls are employed. Androstenediol, for example, with 3β- and 17β-hydroxyl groups cannot be used for the localization of one enzyme in most tissues, since the contribution of the other hydroxyl group cannot be excluded.

B. CHOICE OF STEROID SOLVENT

The ideal solvent for steroid work would be one which dissolved the steroid readily, was usable with buffered aqueous solutions, did not react chemically or physically with any other component of the incubation medium, e.g. Nitro BT, and was not itself a source of hydrogen, thus avoiding problems in controlling reactions. Alcoholic solvents, ethanol, propylene glycol and ethylene glycol, have all been tried but have the disadvantage of themselves acting as a source of hydrogen, aggravating control problems (Ferguson, 1965a, b: Ferguson et al., 1966). Tissues with a high concentration of alcohol dehydrogenase are naturally the most difficult to investigate. Dimethyl formamide has been used with success with most steroids and gives reliable controls. Some recent reports have suggested that this solvent affects the hydrophobic groups of proteins with subsequent changes in enzyme configuration and activity, but the significance of this with respect to the histochemical work is not yet known.

To summarize our experience, propylene glycol was used in all the earlier work, but because of recurrent control difficulty dimethyl formamide is now the solvent of choice.

C. BUFFERS

The choice of buffer does not seem to be of great importance in this histochemical work. In our laboratory veronal, phosphate, Tris HCl and glycylglycine have been used with no detectable differences except that Nitro BT does not remain in solution below pH 6 with phosphate buffer.

D. CO-FACTORS

The dehydrogenation technique depends on NAD or NADP to act as hydrogen-transferring agents between the hydroxysteroid and the final hydrogen acceptor. Nicotinamide has been used in some experimental systems to protect the NAD from enzymic destruction but its value, in our experience, is doubtful. Magnesium ions have often been included in the reaction mixture, but again we have noticed that the addition of small amounts of magnesium did not improve the reaction; with high concentrations of magnesium a degree of inhibition occurred.

E. PHENAZINE METHOSULPHATE

This has been used in enzyme histochemistry as a hydrogen carrier to eliminate diaphorase dependence. Phenazine methosulphate has been used predominantly with succinic dehydrogenase, a flavoprotein-dependent enzyme, and has been found to increase the activity. In this laboratory phenazine methosulphate has been found to be of little value in increasing the reactivity of any of the hydroxysteroid dehydrogenases, and the difficulties attendant on working with phenazine methosulphate make it unsuitable for routine use. Two other quinones have been used as electron carriers in some systems—Vitamin K and ubiquinone—but so far they have not been used extensively in hydroxysteroid dehydrogenase histochemistry.

F. pH

Although biochemical work supplies a wide range of pH optima for the different hydroxysteroid dehydrogenase reactions, we have found that histochemically pH 7-8 is suitable.

G. TETRAZOLIUM SALTS

These salts are used in histochemistry to accept electrons from the oxidized product. Basically the unreduced form of the dye is soluble and the reduced form is insoluble and coloured. The dye in the reduced form is deposited at the site of the enzyme reaction, and it is this fact which makes localization possible. A large number of tetrazolium salts are available for use in histochemical work, each salt having different properties. Some, such as neotetrazolium, are to some extent soluble in the reduced form and the histochemical localization obtained is inferior in this case. Other salts, including the one which has been used predominantly in this laboratory, Nitro Blue Tetrazolium, are extremely insoluble and cannot be removed for quantitative reactions; histochemical localization is however good. Tetranitro BT and MTT cobalt chloride are theoretically suitable alternatives.

The histochemical reaction for the demonstration of the hydroxysteroid dehydrogenases can now be considered in a general form. Briefly, the demonstration depends on the transfer of hydrogen, removed from the hydroxysteroid, via a pyridine nucleotide to a tetrazolium salt which is reduced and deposited at the site of the reaction (Fig. 1). It will be obvious that the reaction depends on the activity of two enzymes, and since the pyridine nucleotides are freely diffusable the localization will ultimately depend on the site of the diaphorase. The accurate localization of hydroxysteroid dehydrogenases then depends on two conditions: (a) that the diaphorase is ubiquitous or at least present in the cells having the hydroxysteroid dehydrogenase, and (b) that the reduced pyridine nucleotides are oxidised rapidly at the site of formation and do not diffuse widely. It is thus important before investigating a new tissue to localize $NADH_2$ and $NADPH_2$ diaphorase lest this be a limiting factor.

The other major problem which concerns the enzymatic component of the system is the solubility of the individual hydroxysteroid dehydrogenases. The definition of a soluble enzyme is difficult in the light of the work of Jones (1965), who showed that up to 70% of protein nitrogen is lost from fresh tissue sections within five minutes of incubation in a phosphate-buffered medium at pH 7. A simplified definition of a soluble enzyme for histochemical work is an enzyme protein which is rapidly and easily removed from unfixed tissue sections, and which can be detected in the incubation medium. (For physicochemical purposes and biochemical work this definition, of course, would be useless.) With the range of enzymes discussed in the review, a large proportion are soluble, particularly 3α-, 17β- and 20α-hydroxysteroid dehydrogenases. Other enzymes, for example 3β- (Rubin and Strecker, 1961) and 11β-hydroxysteroid dehydrogenases (Hurlock and Talalay, 1959), have been shown to be partly soluble and partly insoluble. The problems which this raises are numerous. The most obvious is that a soluble enzyme in the incubation medium may oxidize the steroid and the reduced pyridine nucleotide formed will be oxidized at the site of tetrazolium reductase activity throughout the tissue, and not at the site of the original hydroxysteroid dehydrogenase. Re-use of media following incubation of a tissue will cause contamination of further sections and this is an irresistible argument for individual incubation of tissue sections in fresh solutions.

To surmount the problem of soluble enzymes several techniques have been devised. PVP (Pearse, 1960), gelatin and PVA (Chayen *et al.*, 1965) and Rheomacrodex have been tried, all of which act by increasing the viscosity of the medium and so, theoretically, limiting the diffusion of the proteins. As indicated above, fixation may also be used for this purpose. In our experience, however, localization in fresh frozen sections is sharp and clearcut and the problem of diffusion is more theoretical than actual. Moreover, tissues which have been fixed in formalin vapour or potassium dichromate show the same hydroxysteroid dehydrogenase distribution patterns as fresh tissue. We therefore feel that valid histological conclusions can be drawn from fresh material and that it is feasible to localize enzymes which biochemists would describe as soluble. As examples we would refer the reader to the fresh preparations of mammalian kidney (pp. 126, 128) showing 3α- and 11β-hydroxysteroid dehydrogenases in utterly different situations, despite the 'soluble' nature of both enzymes.

H. PROCEDURE

In summary, the following technical procedure is recommended: the experimental animal is killed and the tissue to be examined immediately removed and frozen. Sections (usually 8–12μ) are cut in a cryostat maintained at −25° C using a cooled knife. The tissue sections are attached to clean, dry, glass coverslips by momentary thawing and allowed to dry. These sections are then incubated separately at 37° C in a buffer medium (pH 7·5) to which NAD or NADP (2 mg/ml), Nitro BT (0·5 mg/ml) and the particular steroid substrate (0·25 mg/ml), dissolved in dimethyl formamide, are added, Control incubations are concurrently carried out with the medium lacking steroid.

IV. POST-INCUBATION TECHNIQUES

On completion of the incubation the sections are thoroughly washed in buffer and water to remove all traces of reagents from the section, leaving only the reduced diformazan, bound to the tissue section. Post-incubation fixation is desirable to halt enzymic reactions capable of reducing the unreduced substantive Nitro BT remaining in the section (Balogh, 1964; Ferguson, 1965c; Wyllie, 1965); 10% formalin in the usual fixative.

Aqueous mountants are used and the slides are examined immediately. Should a delay occur the sections are stored at 4° C in a refrigerator. If unfixed sections are mounted with aqueous mountants continuing reduction of substantive Nitro BT sometimes occurs. Diffusion of formazan into aqueous mounting media, such as Hydramount, occurs over a period of time. Levy *et al.* (1959b) and Kellogg and Glenner (1960) dehydrate their sections prior to examination. Since the pink reaction product, which we accept as evidence of a weak reaction, is removed from the sections by the procedure of washing in alcohol, then trace amounts of activity will be missed. Accordingly, in our view washing in alcohol is not advisable for critical work.

V. ULTRASTRUCTURAL TECHNIQUES

Bradbury and Steward (1964) devised a technique for the ultrastructural demonstration of 3β-hydroxysteroid dehydrogenase. Using hydroxyadipalde-hyde-fixed rat adrenals, small tissue blocks were incubated in the usual medium for five minutes prior to dehydration and sectioning. 3β-Hydroxy-steroid dehydrogenase activity was assigned either to the mitochondrial matrix or to the inner mitochondrial membrane of the fascicular cells. It must be appreciated that in ultrastructural work the final intracellular localization of formazan by this method will depend on the sites of diaphorase activity, and this may or may not correspond to the site of hydroxysteroid dehydrogenase activity. This probably invalidates the use of Nitro BT coupled via diaphorase for ultrastructural investigations and automatically limits the light microscopic conclusions regarding hydroxysteroid dehydro-genase localization to a statement of which cells in a given organ possess the appropriate enzyme, precluding comment on which organelles are the site of activity. The practical significance of this point has already been referred to (p. 5) in relation to acetone washing of sections prior to incubation.

VI. THE HYDROXYSTEROID DEHYDROGENASES

Enzymes which undertake steroid dehydrogenation fall into two broad groups. The first group has been extensively studied in bacteria (Stoudt *et al.*, 1955; Gale *et al.*, 1962; Stefanovic *et al.*, 1963) and accomplishes steroid dehydrogenation by introducing a double bond into the perhydrocyclo-pentenophenanthrene nucleus. This group does not concern us further; suffice it to say that such a hydrogen source is excluded histochemically by incubating tissue sections as controls with the appropriate saturated keto-steroid when investigating the presence of a hydroxysteroid dehydrogenase in the tissue.

The second group of enzymes, the hydroxysteroid dehydrogenases, act by converting an hydroxyl group to the corresponding keto group (Fig. 1), with the removal of two hydrogen atoms. The enzyme is named according to the number of the C-atom in the steroid nucleus (Fig. 3) to which the attacked hydroxyl group is attached; in addition, where relevant, on account of the stereo-specificity of many of the enzymes involved it is necessary to stipulate whether the hydroxyl group dehydrogenated projects above or below the plane of the steroid molecule (Fig. 4). Thus, for example, one encounters a 3α-hydroxysteroid dehydrogenase, a 3β-hydroxysteroid dehydrogenase, a 16α-hydroxysteroid dehydrogenase and a 16β-hydroxysteroid dehydrogenase.

During dehydrogenation of the appropriate hydroxysteroid, the hydroxy-steroid dehydrogenase transfers hydrogen to either NAD or NADP; the

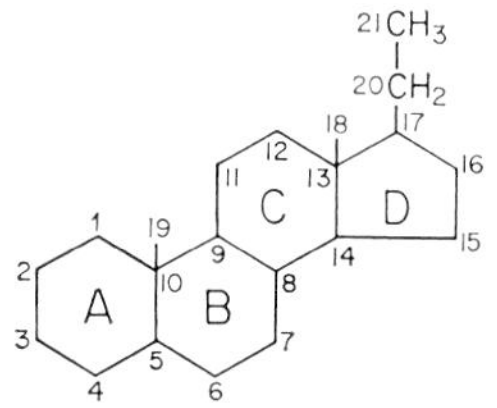

FIG. 3. Illustrative structure showing numbering of carbon atoms and rings in the steroid nucleus.

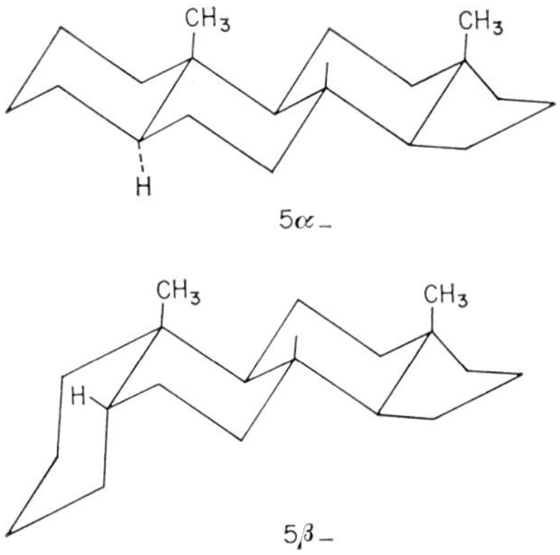

FIG. 4. Indicating the α- and β-positions of the 5-hydrogen on the 5-carbon and their influence on molecular configuration.

pyridine nucleotide specificities of the hydroxysteroid dehydrogenases vary and their requirements in this field will be dealt with separately in relation to each enzyme.

A. 3α-HYDROXYSTEROID DEHYDROGENASE

It seems to be generally agreed that this enzyme, whether obtained from bacterial or mammalian sources, is specific for the 3α-hydroxyl function of 5α- and 5β-steroids. Biochemically it has been noted in the supernatant of rabbit liver and kidney preparations (Ungar and Dorfman, 1954) and has been prepared as an acetone powder from rat liver (Tomkins and Isselbacher, 1954). It is NAD or NADP dependent both biochemically and histochemically.

Dorfman and Ungar (1965) note its occurrence in rat liver, kidney and testis and state that it is absent from spleen, lung, brain and muscle. Histochemically the enzyme will utilize androsterone and aetiocholanolone. In rat ovary corpora lutea a strong 3α-hydroxysteroid dehydrogenase exists which appears to utilize 5α-steroids preferentially.

Biochemically 3α-hydroxysteroid dehydrogenase has been ascribed a trans-hydrogenase function (Fig. 8) (Hurlock and Talalay, 1959), and the presence of 11β-, 17α-, 17β- and 21-hydroxyl groups interferes to a greater or lesser extent with the activity of 3α-hydroxysteroid dehydrogenase (Tomkins and Isselbacher, 1954). Histochemical studies of this sort have not yet been attempted.

B. 3β-HYDROXYSTEROID DEHYDROGENASE

From the biochemist's point of view this is a collective title which includes a Δ^5-3β-hydroxysteroid dehydrogenase, a Δ^4-3β-hydroxysteroid dehydrogenase, 3β-hydroxysteroid dehydrogenase and a 3β (or 17β) -hydroxysteroid dehydrogenase.

The first enzyme, Δ^5-3β-hydroxysteroid dehydrogenase, is concerned with steroid biosynthesis. Testicular, ovarian, adrenal and placental tissues are known biochemically to contain an enzyme complex which irreversibly converts Δ^5-3β-hydroxysteroids to Δ^4-3-ketosteroids (Samuels et al., 1951) and this system is now thought to consist of a Δ^5-3β-hydroxysteroid dehydrogenase together with a Δ^5-Δ^4-ketosteroid isomerase (Fig. 5) (Talalay, 1957).

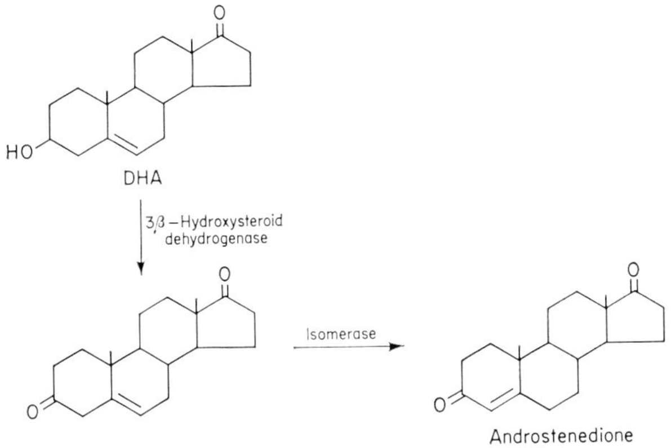

FIG. 5. Illustrating the action of Δ^5-3β-hydroxysteroid dehydrogenase and the appropriate isomerase.

According to Beyer and Samuels (1956), the reaction is NAD mediated, but histochemically (Table 1) a reaction will develop in some tissues with NADP.

The second enzyme, Δ^4-3β-hydroxysteroid dehydrogenase, has not been studied histochemically.

The third enzyme, 3β-hydroxysteroid dehydrogenase, is supposed to act on saturated steroids and to occur in mammalian liver, but its purity and

TABLE 1

		Pregnenolone	3β-Hydroxy-5α-pregnan-20-one	3β-Hydroxy-5β-pregnan-20-one	DHA	3β-Hydroxy-5β-androstan-17-one	3β-Hydroxy-5α-cholestan	3β-Hydroxy-5β-cholestan
Adrenal gland (human, rat, mouse and hamster)	NAD	+	–	+	+++	++++++	–	–
	NADP	tr.	–	–	++	+++	–	–
Testis (human, frog, cock and museum)	NAD	+	–	+	+	+	–	–
	NADP	–	–	–	–	–	–	–
(ram)	NAD	–	–	++	–	tr.	–	–
	NADP	–	–	–	–	–	–	–
Ovary (rat)	NAD	++	–	+	+++	+++++	–	–
	NADP	+	–	+	++	+++	–	–
Placenta (human)	NAD	+	–	++	+++	++++	–	–
	NADP	–	–	+	+	++	–	–
Kidney (rabbit and mouse)	NAD	tr.	–	++	tr.	+++	–	–
	NADP	–	–	+	–	+	–	–
Duodenum (human)	NAD and NADP	–	–	–	–	–	–	–
Preen gland (cockerel)	NAD	–	–	+++	–	+	–	–

This table summarizes our results with various 3β-hydroxysteroids as histochemical substrates. Of particular interest is the fact that Δ⁵-3β-hydroxysteroids give little or no colour reaction in mammalian kidney, avian Leydig cells and avian preen gland, whereas the corresponding 5β-steroids are well utilized. Moreover, although 5β-steroids are well used by most tissues, placental 3β-hydroxysteroid dehydrogenase appears to utilize 5α-steroids as well. The presence of a cholesterol-type sidechain totally impedes histochemical utilization of 3β-hydroxy-5β-steroids.

identification leave much to be desired. It is present in both the particulate and soluble functions and will reduce the 3-ketone of 5α- and 5β-steroids to the 3β-hydroxyl group. Histochemically, Baillie and Mack (1966) and Koide and Mitsudo (1965) have noted a colour reaction in testicular Leydig cells and placental trophoblast, respectively, when incubated with saturated 3β-hydroxysteroids. The histochemical utilization of various saturated 3β-hydroxysteroids has recently been studied in detail in this laboratory and the results are summarized in Table 1.

A study of Table 1 will disclose the following points of biochemical interest. Firstly, saturated 5α-steroids are not utilized vigorously, but 5β-steroids give a strong reaction in many tissues. Secondly, saturated steroids with a cholesterol-type side chain do not undergo dehydrogenation in this histochemical system. Thirdly, several tissues, including ram testis, avian preen gland, rabbit kidney and mammalian liver, exhibit little formazan deposition when incubated with Δ⁵-3β-hydroxysteroids such as DHA but develop massive formazan deposition (Figs. 6 and 7) when incubated with 3β-hydroxy-5β-steroids. These facts fit reasonably well with the known biochemistry of 3β-hydroxysteroid dehydrogenase, but further work is needed to elucidate the interrelationship of 3β-hydroxysteroid dehydrogenase and Δ⁵-3β-hydroxysteroid dehydrogenase, both biochemically and histochemically. The fourth

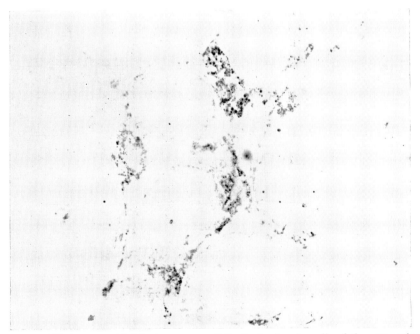

Fɪɢ. 6. 3β-Hydroxysteroid dehydrogenase activity in the Leydig cells of the ram, using 3β-hydroxy-5β-androstan as substrate. No activity is demonstrable in the Leydig cells of this species using Δ⁵-3β-hydroxysteroids such as pregnenolone or DHA. × 180.

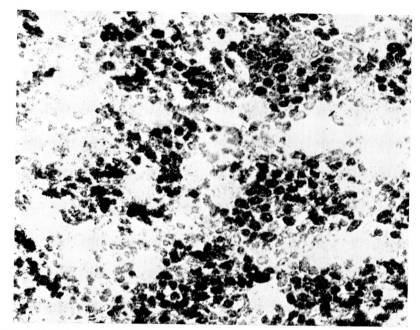

FIG. 7. 3β-Hydroxysteroid dehydrogenase activity in the cortex of the rabbit kidney, using 3β-hydroxy-5β-pregnan-20-one as substrate. Trace Δ⁵-3β-hydroxysteroid dehydrogenase activity only is demonstrable in this kidney, using Δ⁵-3β-hydroxysteroids as substrate. × 70.

enzyme of the group, the 3(or 17)β-hydroxysteroid dehydrogenase is bacterial in origin and somewhat non-specific. It seems likely that the first three enzymes of this group, which are mammalian in origin, are much more rigidly specific (Dorfman and Ungar, 1965).

C. 6β-HYDROXYSTEROID DEHYDROGENASE

Little work has been done on this enzyme and its existence has been inferred from naturally occurring steroids and reaction products.

D. 11β-HYDROXYSTEROID DEHYDROGENASE

Biochemically this enzyme has been demonstrated in liver, kidney, testis and placenta, and will utilize either NAD or NADP (Hubener et al., 1956; Hurlock and Talalay, 1959; Mahesh and Ulrich, 1959; Osinski, 1960). Biochemically and histochemically it shows low substrate specificity. 11β-Hydroxyandrostenedione is the histochemical substrate of choice.

E. 16α- AND 16β-HYDROXYSTEROID DEHYDROGENASES

These enzymes are poorly documented biochemically. Histochemically

NAD is the usual co-factor in human testis; adrenal, ovary and placental 16β-hydroxysteroid dehydrogenase will also use NADP, and an aromatic A-ring configuration is less well utilized than a Δ^5 A-ring configuration.

F. 17β-HYDROXYSTEROID DEHYDROGENASE

In the placenta a 17β-hydroxysteroid dehydrogenase, which is specific for the 17β-hydroxyl function of steroids with an aromatic A-ring, has been studied biochemically (Langer *et al.*, 1959; Adams *et al.*, 1962; Jarabak *et al.*, 1962, 1963). In the avian preen gland a testosterone-specific 17β-hydroxysteroid dehydrogenase occurs histochemically; there is therefore evidence for at least two stereo-specific 17β-hydroxysteroid dehydrogenases. Both will dehydrogenate saturated A-ring steroids, the 5α-configuration being better used (cf. 3β-hydroxysteroid dehydrogenase).

G. 20α- AND 20β-HYDROXYSTEROID DEHYDROGENASE

20α-Hydroxysteroid dehydrogenase is responsible for the interconversions of 20α-hydroxyprogesterone with progesterone (Wiest, 1959; Wiest and Wilcox, 1961), and is considered biochemically to use NADP as co-factor. Information about 20β-hydroxysteroid dehydrogenase, on the other hand, is scant and in the histochemical system appears to be NAD dependent.

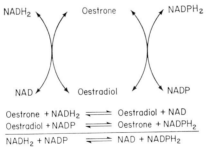

$$Oestrone + NADH_2 \rightleftharpoons Oestradiol + NAD$$
$$Oestradiol + NADP \rightleftharpoons Oestrone + NADPH_2$$
$$\overline{NADH_2 + NADP \rightleftharpoons NAD + NADPH_2}$$

FIG. 8. The diagram and equation illustrate the meaning of a transhydrogenase reaction; by this means hydrogen is transferred from cellular enzyme systems requiring NAD as co-factor to those requiring NADP, or vice versa.

VII. METABOLIC PATHWAYS OF STEROIDS

The particular pathways considered at this point will be dealt with in greater detail where relevant in the sections concerning the tissues which have been examined. An initial consideration of general steroid metabolic pathways is desirable to place the succeeding results in perspective. For convenience steroid metabolism can be divided into the following stages: (1) cholesterol synthesis, (2) pregnenolone synthesis and metabolism, (3) progesterone metabolism, (4) corticosteroid synthesis and metabolism, (5) androgen synthesis and metabolism, (6) oestrogen synthesis and metabolism. Many of these pathways overlap but this artificial division is convenient.

A. CHOLESTEROL SYNTHESIS

Only one step between acetate and cholesterol is amenable to demonstration by a histochemical dehydrogenase technique. This is the oxidation of the 3β-hydroxy to the 3-keto group of norlanosterol converting it to $\Delta^{8,24}$-4,4-dimethylcholestadiene-3-one. This step seems to be necessary before the removal of the two methyl groups at the 4-position (Bloch, 1959).

The sequence of reactions leading to the formation of cholesterol are summarized in Figure 9. (Popjak *et al.*, 1962).

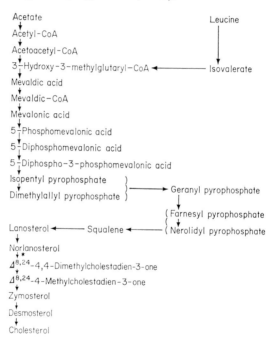

FIG. 9. Scheme of cholesterol biosynthesis. * Indicates site of action of 3β-hydroxysteroid dehydrogenase.

B. PREGNENOLONE SYNTHESIS AND METABOLISM

Pathways from cholesterol to C_{21} derivatives involve scission of the side chain to form pregnenolone and isocaproic acid (Shimizu *et al.*, 1961).

The mechanism of this cleavage has been investigated, and it is established that 20α-cholesterol is an intermediate and that 20α, 22ξ-dihydroxycholesterol is also involved. Shimizu *et al.* (1962) suggest that the intermediate 20α-hydroxy-22-ketocholesterol is on the metabolic pathway, implying that a dehydrogenation is involved. Other workers (Constantopoulous *et al.*, 1962), however, using 20α-hydroxycholesterol analogues lacking 22-keto groups, found that these were also converted to pregnenolone. This pathway cannot yet be tackled histochemically.

Pregnenolone, once formed, may be converted to progesterone by a Δ⁵-3β-hydroxysteroid dehydrogenase or to 17α-hydroxypregnenolone and DHA, as indicated in Fig. 10.

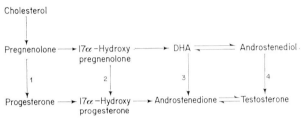

FIG. 10. Δ⁵-3β-Hydroxysteroid dehydrogenase catalyses reactions 1–4.

C. PROGESTERONE METABOLISM

Progesterone is a precursor of corticosteroids, androgens and oestrogens. 20α- and 20β-hydroxy derivatives of progesterone are known, implying the existence of 20α- and 20β-hydroxysteroid dehydrogenases. Figure 11 briefly outlines the major metabolic pathways of progesterone.

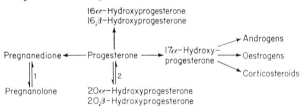

FIG. 11. A scheme of progesterone metabolism. 3α-Hydroxysteroid dehydrogenase is responsible for conversion 1, 20α- and 20β-hydroxysteroid dehydrogenases for conversion 2.

D. CORTICOSTEROID SYNTHESIS AND METABOLISM

This is an extremely complex area of steroid metabolism, and only those pathways which appear relevant in the present context will be mentioned.

The initial step is the conversion of the Δ⁵-3β-hydroxyl group of pregnenolone to a Δ⁴-3 keto group which can be demonstrated histochemically. The next series of steps involves hydroxylation reactions successively at positions 17α, 21 and 11β to form cortisol, or at positions 21 and 11β to form corticosterone (Fig. 12). So far none of these hydroxylation reactions has been histochemically demonstrated.

The further metabolism of these compounds also involves hydroxysteroid dehydrogenases. Thus excretion of cortisol is in the form of dihydro- and

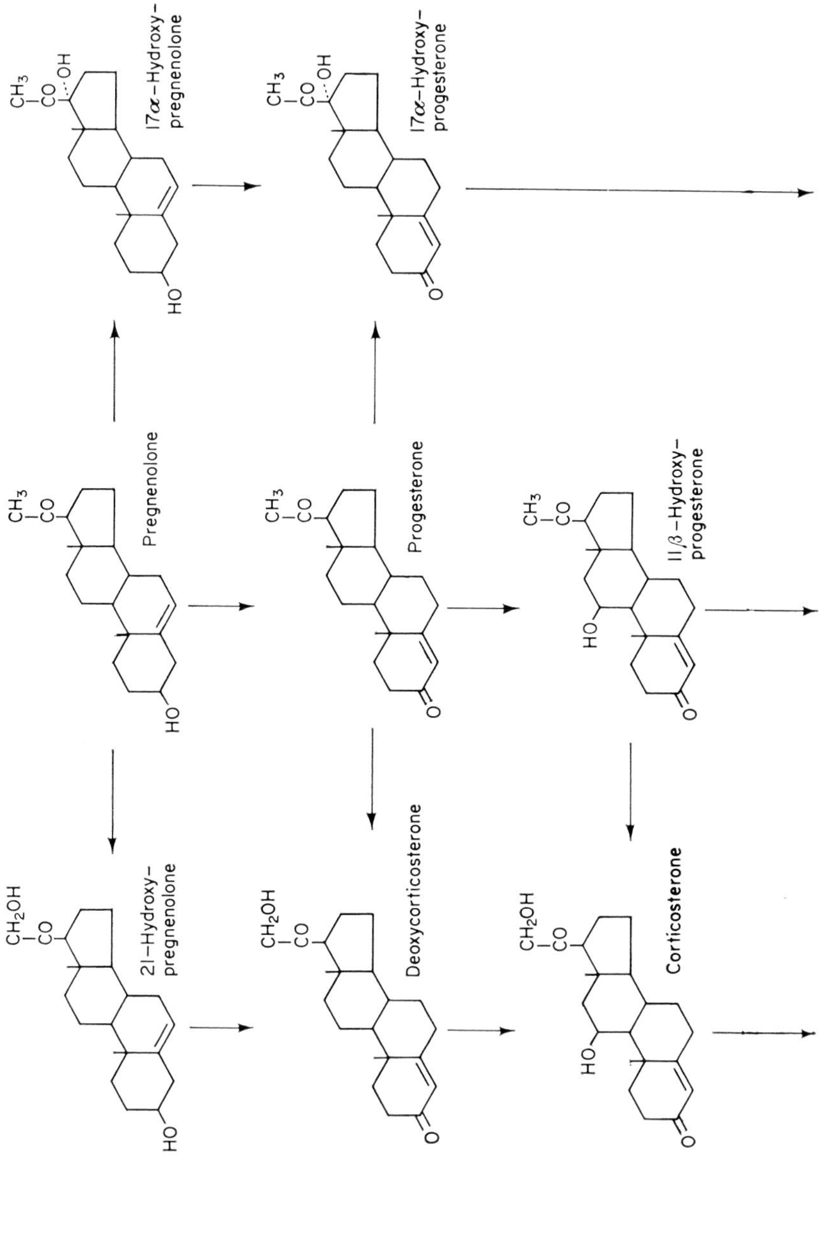
17α–Hydroxy-pregnenolone
17α–Hydroxy-progesterone
Pregnenolone
Progesterone
11β–Hydroxy-progesterone
21–Hydroxy-pregnenolone
Deoxycorticosterone
Corticosterone

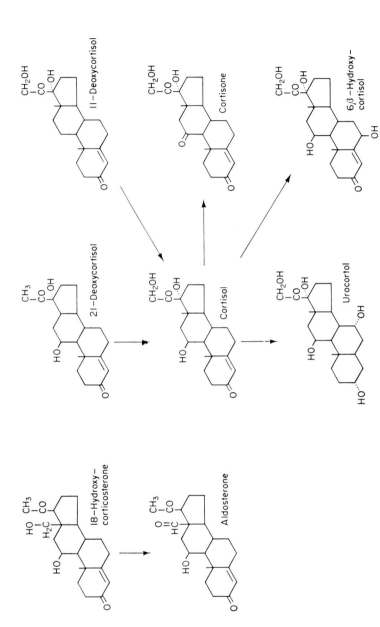

Fig. 12. Scheme of corticosteroid biosynthesis and metabolism.

tetrahydro-3α-hydroxy derivatives. Similarly, both cortisol and corticosterone may undergo dehydrogenation at the 11β-position. The 20-keto group may also be reduced, and Lambert and Pennington (1964) have isolated 20β-hydroxy derivatives of 6β-hydroxy cortisol, implying a 20β-hydroxysteroid dehydrogenase; similarly, Vermulen and Caspi (1958) have isolated 20α- and 20β-hydroxy derivatives in the urine of patients given prednisolone. These reactions are summarized in Fig. 12.

E. ANDROGEN BIOSYNTHESIS AND METABOLISM

This area of steroid metabolism has recently been extensively reviewed (Dorfman et al., 1963). The biosynthesis of androgens occurs by a variety of mechanisms, and in the majority a hydroxysteroid dehydrogenase plays some part, so that the site of these reactions can be localized (Fig. 40).

F. OESTROGEN METABOLISM

The biosynthesis of oestrogens is an extremely active field of steroid research. Essentially the process involves the conversion of a C_{19} compound with a Δ^4-3 keto group, to a C_{18} compound with an aromatic A-ring. Androstenedione and testosterone are precursors, and the first step in the reaction is believed to be the hydroxylation of the C_{19} methyl group. The subsequent steps involve the removal of the hydroxymethyl group, and two possible mechanisms exist for this reaction (Engel, 1959). First, there is dehydrogenation of the hydroxymethyl group to an aldehyde, then to a carboxyl group, with subsequent decarboxylation. The second pathway involves the liberation of the hydroxymethyl group directly as a C_1 fragment.

Once formed, oestrogens undergo a series of oxidation and reduction reactions, amenable to histochemical detection. Initially there is the oestradiol–oestrone interconversion followed by oxidation and reduction at the 16 oxygen function. 6α- and 6β-hydroxy derivatives of oestrogens are interconverted via the 6-keto derivative (Breuer et al., 1958). Reference to Figs. 52 and 53 (Chapter 5) illustrates the metabolism of oestrogens.

VIII. SPECIFICITY CONSIDERATIONS

The interpretation to be placed on the histochemical results obtained with hydroxysteroid dehydrogenase techniques depends on specificity. In our view there are eight reasons for believing that the techniques demonstrate separate substrate-specific enzymes.

A. BIOCHEMICAL OBSERVATIONS

As indicated above in the paragraphs on the individual hydroxysteroid dehydrogenases, most biochemists accept that such mammalian hydroxysteroid dehydrogenases as have been isolated and characterized biochemically are specific for a particular hydroxyl group, for example 3β-hydroxysteroid dehydrogenase (Samuels *et al.*, 1951) and 17β-hydroxysteroid dehydrogenase (Jarabak *et al.*, 1962). It would be reasonable to expect that enzymes which are highly stereo-specific biochemically would behave similarly in tissue sections.

B. TISSUE DISTRIBUTION OF HYDROXYSTEROID DEHYDROGENASES

In the light of recent observations it is possible to point to several tissues which possess only one hydroxysteroid dehydrogenase. For example, human duodenal mucosa possesses 17β-hydroxysteroid dehydrogenase activity only; human renal collecting tubules possess 11β-hydroxysteroid dehydrogenase only; the human zona glomerulosa possesses intense 16β-hydroxysteroid dehydrogenase activity, poor Δ^5-3β-hydroxysteroid dehydrogenase activity and no other obvious hydroxysteroid dehydrogenases. In lower animals equally striking examples of selective tissue localization exist. For instance, in rat ovary 17β-hydroxysteroid dehydrogenase occurs only in the germinal epithelium and 20α-hydroxysteroid dehydrogenase is virtually confined to the corpora lutea of the rat ovary. In the hamster adrenal most hydroxysteroid dehydrogenases, including 3β- and 16β-hydroxysteroid dehydrogenases, are evenly distributed throughout the cortex, whereas 11β-hydroxysteroid dehydrogenase is restricted to the inner half or so of the cortex.

C. PYRIDINE NUCLEOTIDE REQUIREMENTS

Hydroxysteroid dehydrogenases both histochemically and biochemically fall into three groups: (*a*) enzymes which are predominantly NAD dependent, such as 3β- and 20β-hydroxysteroid dehydrogenases, (*b*) enzymes which utilize both NAD and NADP well, for example 3α- and 17β-hydroxysteroid dehydrogenases, and (*c*) NADP-dependent enzymes such as 20α-hydroxy-steroid dehydrogenase (Hurlock and Talalay, 1959; Jarabak *et al.*, 1962; Balogh, 1964). Further work is required on this topic.

D. BEHAVIOUR OF DIFFERENT STEREOISOMERS

11α- And 17α-hydroxysteroids are not used to any extent by any tissue, whereas 11β- and 17β-hydroxysteroids give a moderate or intense reaction in tissues such as kidney and placenta. Steric hindrance may play a part in these results. A more subtle, but equally important, difference between stereoisomers is the fact that the histochemical reaction may vary in its pyridine nucleotide requirements. Thus 20α-hydroxysteroid dehydrogenase uses NADP well histochemically, whereas 20β-hydroxysteroid dehydrogenase is predominantly NAD dependent in most tissues.

E. SEX DIFFERENCES

Hepatic (Chapter 10) hydroxysteroid dehydrogenase activity shows pro-nounced sex differences both histochemically and biochemically.

F. INFLUENCE OF MOLECULAR MORPHOLOGY ON HYDROXYSTEROID DEHYDROGENASE ACTIVITY

In the human placental trophoblast the 17β-hydroxysteroid dehydrogenase is specific for aromatic 17β-hydroxysteroids, and in the avian preen gland the 17β-hydroxysteroid dehydrogenase present is almost specific for 17β-hydroxysteroids with a Δ^4-3-keto A-ring configuration. Similarly, in the rodent corpora lutea 3α-hydroxysteroids with a 5α-configuration are well used, whereas 5β-steroids are poorly utilized; by contrast, the saturated 3β-hydroxysteroids behave in the opposite manner in rat corpora lutea. Thus a poor reaction develops with the 5α-3β-hydroxysteroids, whereas those with a 5β-configuration give a massive histochemical reaction.

G. SPECIES VARIATION

Fine differences occur in every organ's pattern of hydroxysteroid dehydrogenase activity, and this is perhaps best shown (Chapter 7) in the phylogenetic development of mesonephric and metanephric hydroxysteroid dehydrogenases.

H. AGE CHANGES

As indicated in Chapters 4 and 5, progressive maturation and development of the gonads is characterized by progressive acquisition of different hydroxysteroid dehydrogenases at different ages.

I. CONCLUSION

The simplest explanation of all these findings is that hydroxysteroid dehydrogenases are specific in these histochemical conditions, and we prefer this view to other possible explanations, including those based on membrane permeability factors and non-specific alcohol dehydrogenases. Any alternative hypothesis must adequately account for *all* the points established above.

REFERENCES

Adams, J. A., Jarabak, J. and Talalay, P. (1962). The steroid specificity of the 17β-hydroxysteroid dehydrogenase of human placenta. *J. Biol. Chem.* **237**, 3067–3073.

Baillie, A. H. and Mack, W. S. (1966). Hydroxysteroid dehydrogenases in normal and abnormal human testes. *J. Endocrinol.* **35**, 239–248.

Baillie, A. H., Calman, K. C., Ferguson, M. M. and Hart, D. McK. (1965a). Histochemical demonstration of 20β-hydroxysteroid dehydrogenase. *J. Endocrinol.* **32**, 337–339.

Baillie, A. H., Calman, K. C., Ferguson, M. M. and Hart, D. McK. (1966a). Histochemical utilisation of 3α-, 6β-, 11α-, 12α-, 16α-, 16β-, 17α-, 21- and 24-hydroxysteroids. *J. Endocrinol.* **34**, 1–12.

Baillie, A. H., Calman, K. C., Ferguson, M. M. and Hart, D. McK. (1966b).

Histochemical distribution of hydroxysteroid dehydrogenases in kidney and liver. *Histochemie* (5, 384-395).

Baillie, A. H., Ferguson, M. M., Calman, K. C. and Hart, D. McK. (1965b). Histochemical demonstration of 11β-hydroxysteroid dehydrogenase. *J. Endocrinol.* 33, 119–125.

Balogh, K. (1964). A histochemical method for the demonstration of 20α-hydroxysteroid dehydrogenase activity in rat ovaries. *J. Histochem. Cytochem.* 12, 670–673.

Bell, L. G. E. (1952). Cooling bath for cytological investigations. *Nature* 170, 719.

Beyer, K. F. and Samuels, L. T. (1956). Distribution of steroid-3β-ol dehydrogenase in cellular structures of the adrenal gland. *J. Biol. Chem.* 219, 69.

Bitensky, L., Lynch, R., Silcox, A. A. and Chayen, J. (1965). Studies on chilling and sectioning tissue for histochemistry. *J. Roy. Microscop. Soc.* 84, 397–398.

Bloch, K. (1959). In: *Biosynthesis of Terpenes and Sterols.* Ed. G. E. W. Wolstenholme, p. 4 (Churchill, London).

Bradbury, S. and Steward, V. W. (1964). A note on the electron staining of diformazan deposits in tissue sections. *J. Roy. Microscop. Soc.* 83, 467–470.

Breuer, H., Nocke, L. and Knuppen, R. (1958). 6β-Hydroxylierung von Oestrogenen in der Rattenleber. *Naturwissenschaften* 45, 397.

Chayen, J., Wells, P. A. and Bitensky, L. (1965). The meaning of a 'good' histochemical reaction in relation to the problem of latent enzyme activity. *J. Roy. Microscop. Soc.* 84, 400–401.

Constantopoulos, G., Satoh, P. S. and Tchen, T. T. (1962). Cleavage of cholesterol side chain by adrenal cortex. III. Identification of 20α, 22-dihydroxycholesterol as an intermediate. *Biochem. Biophys. Res. Communs* 81, 50–55.

Dawson, I. M. P., Pryse-Davies, J. and Snape, I. M. (1961). The histochemical demonstration of steroid 3β-ol dehydrogenase and diphosphopyridine nucleotide diaphorase in the adrenal cortex. *Biochem J.* 78, 16p.

Deane, H. W., Lobel, B. L. and Romney, S. L. (1962). Enzyme histochemistry of normal ovaries of the menstrual cycle, pregnancy and early puerperium. *Am. J. Obstet. Gynecol.* 83, 281–294.

Dorfman, R. I. and Ungar, F. (1965). *Metabolism of steroid hormones* (Academic Press, New York).

Dorfman, R. I., Forchielli, E. and Gut, M. (1963). Unpublished data—quoted from Dorfman and Ungar (1965).

Engel, L. L. (1959). The biosynthesis of estrogens. *Cancer* 10, 711–715.

Ferguson, M. M. (1965a). Observations on the histochemical distribution of alcohol dehydrogenase. *Quart. J. Microscop. Sci.* 106, 289–297.

Ferguson, M. M. (1965b). Histochemical observations on alcohol dehydrogenase. *J. Roy. Microscop. Soc.* 84, 403.

Ferguson, M. M. (1965c). 3β-Hydroxysteroid dehydrogenase activity in the mouse ovary. *J. Endocrinol.* 32, 365–371.

Ferguson, M. M., Baillie, A. H., Calman, K. C. and Hart, D. McK. (1966). The histochemical distribution of alcohol dehydrogenase in endocrine tissues. *Nature* (210, 1277-1279).

Fuhrmann, K. (1961). Uber den histochemischen Nachweis der 3β-ol-Steroiddehydrogenase-Aktivitat in Geweben endokriner Organe. *Zentr. Gynaekol.* 15, 565–572.

Gale, P. H., Page, A. C., Stoudt, T. H. and Folkers, K. (1962). Identification of vitamin K2 (35), an apparent cofactor of a steroidal Δ'-dehydrogenase of Bacillus sphaericus. *Biochemistry*, 1, 788–792.

Hagerman, D. D. and Villee, C. A. (1952). The transport of fructose by human placenta. *J. Clin. Invest.* **31**, 911–913.

Hagerman, D. D. and Villee, C. A. (1953). Effects of the menstrual cycle on the metabolism of human endometrium. *Endocrinology* **53**, 667–673.

Hart, D. McK., Baillie, A. H., Calman, K. C. and Ferguson, M. M. (1966). Hydroxysteroid dehydrogenase development in mouse adrenal and gonads. *J. Anat. (London)* (in press).

Hoerr, N. L. (1936). Cytological studies by the Altmann-Gersh freezing-drying method. I. Recent advances in the technique. *Anat. Record* **65**, 293–317.

Hubener, H. J., Fukushima, D. and Gallagher, T. F. (1956). Substrate specificity of enzymes reducing the 11- and 20-keto groups of steroids. *J. Biol. Chem.* **220**, 499–511.

Hurlock, B. and Talalay, P. (1959). Microsomal 3α- and 11β-hydroxysteroid dehydrogenases. *Arch. Biochem. Biophys.* **80**, 468–9.

Ikonen, M., Niemi, M., Pesonen, S. and Timonen, S. (1961). Histochemical localization of four dehydrogenase systems in the human ovary during the menstrual cycle. *Acta Endocrinol.* **38**, 293–302.

Jarabak, J., Adams, J. A. and Talalay, P. (1962). Purification of a 17β-hydroxysteroid dehydrogenase of human placenta and studies on its transhydrogenase function. *J. Biol. Chem.* **237**, 345–357.

Jarabak, J., Adams, J. A. and Talalay, P. (1963). Properties of 17β-hydroxysteroid dehydrogenase of human placenta. *Federation Proc.* **22**, 468.

Jones, G. R. N. (1965). Losses of nitrogenous material occurring from fresh frozen section during incubation. *J. Roy. Microscop. Soc.* **84**, 399.

Kellogg, D. A. and Glenner, G. G. (1960). Histochemical localisation of human term placental 17β-oestradiol dehydrogenases. Implications for transhydrogenase reaction. *Nature* **187**, 763–764.

Koide, S. S. and Mitsudo, S. M. (1965). Histochemical study of 3β- and 17β-hydroxysteroid dehydrogenases in human term placenta. *Endocrinology* **79**, 403–406.

Kormano, M., Harkonen, M. and Kontinen, E. (1964). Effect of experimental cryptorchidism on the histochemically demonstrable dehydrogenases of the rat testes. *Endocrinology* **74**, 44–51.

Lambert, M. and Pennington, G. W. (1964). Isolation and identification of 20β-hydroxy derivatives of 6β-hydroxycortisol and 6β-hydroxycortisone. *Nature* **203**, 656.

Langer, L. J., Alexander, J. A. and Engel, L. L. (1959). Human placental estradiol-17β dehydrogenase. II. Kinetics and substrate specificities. *J. Biol. Chem.* **234**, 2609–2614.

Levy, H., Deane, H. W. and Rubin, B. L. (1959a). Observations on steroid 3β-ol dehydrogenase activity in steroid-producing glands. *J. Histochem. Cytochem.* **7**, 320.

Levy, H., Deane, H. W. and Rubin, B. L. (1959b). Visualisation of steroid 3β-ol dehydrogenase activity in tissues of intact and hypophysectomised rats. *Endocrinology* **65**, 932–943.

Mahesh, V. B. and Ulrich, F. (1959). Distribution of enzyme systems responsible for steroid metabolism in different tissues and subcellular fractions. *Nature* **184**, 1147–1148.

Marx, A. J., Deane, H. W., Mowles, T. F. and Sheppard, H. (1963). Chronic administration of angiotensin in rats; changes in blood pressure, renal and adrenal histophysiology and aldosterone production. *Endocrinology* 73, 329–337.

Osinski, P. A. (1960). Steroid 11β-ol dehydrogenase in human placenta. *Nature* **187**, 777.

Pearse, A. G. E. (1960). *Histochemistry, theoretical and applied* (Churchill, London).

Pearson, B. and Grose, F. (1959a). Histochemical study of some DPNH and DPN dependent dehydrogenases. *Federation Proc.* **18**, 499.

Pearson, B. and Grose, F. (1959b). Histochemical demonstration of 17β-hydroxy-steroid dehydrogenase by use of a tetrazolium salt. *Proc. Soc. Exptl. Biol. Med.* **100**, 636–638.

Popjak, G., Cornforth, J. W., Cornforth, R. H., Ryhage, R. and Goodman, de W. S. (1962). Studies on the biosynthesis of cholesterol. XVI. Chemical synthesis of $1\text{-}H^3\text{-}2\text{-}C^{14}$ and $1\text{-}D_2\text{-}2\text{-}C^{14}$-trans-farnesyl pyrophosphate and their utilization in squalene biosynthesis. *J. Biol. Chem.* **237**, 56–61.

Rubin, B. L., Deane, H. W. and Hamilton, J. A. (1963a). Biochemical and histo-chemical studies on $\Delta^5\text{-}3\beta$-hydroxysteroid dehydrogenase activity in the adrenal glands and ovaries of diverse mammals. *Endocrinology* **73**, 748–763.

Rubin, B. L., Deane, H. W., Hamilton, J. A. and Driks, E. C. (1963b). Changes in $\Delta^5\text{-}3\beta$-hydroxysteroid dehydrogenase activity in the ovaries of maturing rats. *Endocrinology* **72**, 924–930.

Rubin, B. L. and Strecker, H. J. (1961). Further studies on the sex-influenced activity of 3β-hydroxysteroid dehydrogenase of rat liver. *Endocrinology* **72**, 764–770.

Samuels, L., Helmrich, M., Lasater, M. and Reich, H. (1951). An enzyme in endo-crine tissues which oxidises $\Delta^5\text{-}3\beta$-hydroxysteroids to unsaturated ketones. *Science* **113**, 440.

Scott, G. H. (1933). A critical study and review of the method of micro-incineration. *Protoplasma* **20**, 133–151.

Shimizu, K., Gut, M. and Dorfman, R. I. (1962). 20, 22-Di-hydroxycholesterol, a intermediate in the biosynthesis of pregnenolone (3β-hydroxypregn-5-en-20-one) from cholesterol. *J. Biol. Chem.* **237**, 699–702.

Shimizu, K., Hayano, M., Gut, M. and Dorfman, R. I. (1961). The transformation of 20α-hydroxycholesterol to isocaproic acid and C21 steroids. *J. Biol. Chem.* **236**, 695–699.

Stefanovic, V., Hayano, M. and Dorfman, R. I. (1963). Some observations on the Δ^1-dehydrogenation of steroids by *Bacillus sphaericus*. *Biochim. Biophys. Acta* **71**, 429–437.

Stoudt, T. H., McAleer, W. J., Chemerola, J. M., Kozlowski, M. A. Hirschmann, R. F., Marlatt, V. and Miller, R. (1955). The microbial 1-dehydro-genation of some Δ^1-3-keto-steroids. *Arch. Biochem. Biophys.* **59**, 304–305.

Talalay, P. (1957). Enzymatic mechanisms in steroid metabolism. *Physiol. Rev.* **37**, 362–389.

Talalay, P. (1965). Enzymatic mechanisms in steroid biochemistry. *Ann. Rev. Biochem* **34**, 347–380

Talalay, P and Williams-Ashman, H. G. (1960) Participation of steroid hormones in the enzymatic transfer of hydrogen. *Record Progr. Hormone Res.* **16**, 1–47.

Tomkins, G. M. and Isselbacher, K. J. (1954). Enzymic reduction of cortisone. *J. Am. Chem. Soc.* **76**, 3100–3101.

Ungar, F. and Dorfman, R. I. (1954). The conversion of 17α, 21-dihydroxypregnane-3, 20-dione to 3α, 17α, 21-tri-hydroxypregnan-20-one. *J. Am. Chem. Soc.* **76**, 1197–1198.

B

Vermulen, A. and Caspi, E. (1958). The metabolism of prednisolone by homogenates of rat liver. *J. Biol. Chem.* **233**, 54–56.

Wattenberg, L. W. (1958). Microscopic histochemical demonstration of steroid-3β-ol dehydrogenase in tissue sections. *J. Histochem. Cytochem.* **6**, 225–232.

Wiest, W. G. (1959). Conversion of progesterone to 4-pregnen-20α-ol-3-one by rat ovarian tissue in vitro. *J. Biol. Chem.* **234**, 3115–3121.

Wiest, W. G. and Wilcox, R. B. (1961). Purification and properties of rat ovarian 20α-hydroxysteroid dehydrogenase. *J. Biol. Chem.* **236**, 2425–2428.

Wyllie, R. G. (1965). Fixation in enzyme histochemistry. *Nature* **207**, 93–4.

CHAPTER 2

The Sebaceous and Preen Glands

I. HUMAN SEBACEOUS GLANDS

In a preliminary study of human skin (Baillie *et al.*, 1965), no evidence of significant hydroxysteroid dehydrogenase activity was noted in the epidermis, dermis, hair follicles or sweat glands, although considerable difficulty was being experienced in controlling epidermis and hair shafts, apparently because of the presence of some factor in these tissues which spontaneously reduced Nitro BT and which can be destroyed by boiling.

Baillie *et al.* (1965) established a significant morphological difference between the sebaceous glands from areas prone to acne vulgaris and those in other parts of the body; strong Δ^5-3β-, 16β- and 17β-hydroxysteroid dehydrogenase activity and moderate or weak 3α- and 11β-hydroxysteroid dehydrogenase activity is demonstrable in sebaceous glands from the upper part of the back. No hydroxysteroid dehydrogenase activity is present in the sebaceous glands of the forearm or lower limb.

In order to test this apparent link between the clinical incidence of acne vulgaris and sebaceous gland hydroxysteroid dehydrogenase activity, a full study of nearly 150 full thickness skin biopsies followed (Baillie *et al.*, 1966).

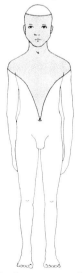

FIG. 13. Anatomical distribution of sebaceous glands exhibiting histochemically demonstrable hydroxysteroid dehydrogenase activity.

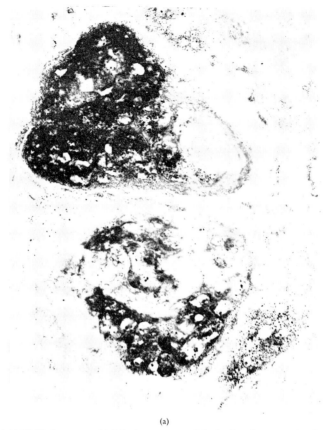

(a)

FIG. 14. (a) Δ^5-3β-Hydroxysteroid dehydrogenase activity in the sebaceous glands of a biopsy from the face of a 15-year-old girl. DHA was the substrate chosen. × 100.

In man, sebaceous glands are distributed throughout the skin, except the palms of the hands, the soles of the feet and the lower lip. They vary in size and number with the individual, site and age, but are most numerous on the scalp, where they may number 900 glands per square centimetre of skin. Over the remainder of the skin surface there are usually fewer than 100 glands per square centimetre.

Sebaceous glands with histochemically demonstrable hydroxysteroid dehydrogenase activity occur on the face, nose, forehead, cheeks, neck, back, anterior chest wall and epigastric areas (Baillie *et al.*, 1966); hydroxysteroid dehydrogenase activity is lacking in sebaceous glands of the arm (except over the deltoid area), forearm, dorsum of hand, hypogastric and iliac areas, and from those of the lower limb (Fig. 13). In those glands exhibiting hydroxysteroid dehydrogenase activity the reaction product is deposited as minute granules of diformazan throughout the cells of the sebaceous gland (Fig. 14).

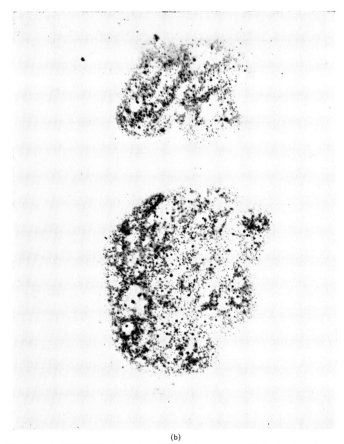

(b)

FIG. 14. Continued. (b) 17β-Hydroxysteroid dehydrogenase activity in the sebaceous glands of a biopsy from the scapular area of a 28-year-old male. Testosterone was the substrate chosen. $\times 90$.

Little or no formazan is seen in sebaceous gland lipids.

Although Baillie *et al.* (1966) failed to note any sex difference in the distribution of hydroxysteroid dehydrogenases in human sebaceous glands, quite marked age changes were observed (Fig. 15). Activity is maximal during the first two decades of life and progressively falls off thereafter with advancing age.

The function of 3α-, Δ^5-3β-, 11β-, 16β- and 17β-hydroxysteroid dehydrogenases in steroid biosynthesis and excretion in organs such as adrenal, gonad and kidney is reasonably well understood; the physiological role of these enzymes in the sebaceous glands is unclear (see below) and it seems unlikely that they are related to cholesterol or vitamin D synthesis.

The important point is that the anatomical distribution of hydroxysteroid dehydrogenase-containing sebaceous glands strikingly resembles the clinical

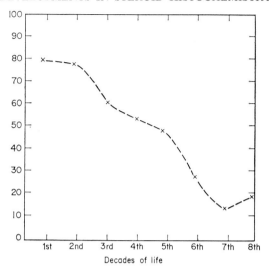

Fɪɢ. 15. A crude quantitation of the drop in activity noted in sebaceous gland hydroxysteroid
dehydrogenases with age.

distribution of acne vulgaris. Thus the scalp, for example, is virtually never
involved in acne vulgaris and even in the severest forms the lesions do not
extend beyond the scalp margins; its sebaceous glands do not exhibit hydroxysteroid dehydrogenase activity. In the same way acne vulgaris lesions occur
on the face, neck, upper part of trunk and lateral aspect of arm, that is, in just
those areas whose sebaceous glands exhibit hydroxysteroid dehydrogenase
activity. Moreover, the quantitative decline in hydroxysteroid dehydrogenase
activity (Fig. 15) with age parallels the clinical improvement of acne. In this
context the presence of sebaceous gland hydroxysteroid dehydrogenases from
birth is at variance with the clinical observation that acne usually initially
appears at puberty, but it must be borne in mind that acne is a complex
disease, which is profoundly affected by the sex hormones and corticosteroids
(Strauss and Pochi, 1963).

In particular, androgens such as testosterone have been shown (Strauss *et
al.*, 1962; Pochi *et al.*, 1963) to stimulate sebaceous gland activity in man,
and in human castrates sebaceous activity can be partly sustained (Pochi *et al.*,
1962) by steroids of adrenal origin. DHA appears to be the principal adrenal
androgen involved (Pochi *et al.*, 1963) in sebaceous gland stimulation, and
glucocorticoids are supposed to act in a permissive capacity facilitating
sebaceous gland response to DHA. In these circumstances the existence of a
Δ^5-3β-hydroxysteroid dehydrogenase and a 17β-hydroxysteroid dehydrogenase in the sebaceous glands prone to acne vulgaris is of especial interest
since it indicates that these glands selectively have the ability to further
metabolize the steroids (DHA and testosterone) which stimulate them.
Preliminary biochemical work has established a substantially greater con-

version rate from DHA to testosterone in skin from human shoulder compared with skin from thigh (Cameron *et al.*, 1966).

Whereas androgens stimulate sebaceous gland secretion and aggravate acne, oestrogens tend to have the reverse effect, causing atrophy of the sebaceous glands. In this context it is interesting to note that several biochemical workers have encountered a degree of inhibition of hydroxysteroid dehydrogenases by aromatic or phenolic steroids of the oestrogen type. The histochemical observations in human sebaceous glands not only fit well the clinical distribution of acne vulgaris, but also offer a possible explanation of the effects of androgens and oestrogens on the sebaceous glands.

Although the evidence is circumstantial, it seems fair to conclude that sebaceous gland hydroxysteroid dehydrogenases play a part in acne vulgaris, but much remains to be done to elucidate their role.

II. SEBACEOUS GLANDS OR THEIR EQUIVALENT IN LOWER ANIMALS

In the mouse and rat (A. H. Baillie, unpublished observation) no sebaceous glands exhibit any hydroxysteroid dehydrogenase activity. Since these animals do not suffer from acne vulgaris, this could be construed as further evidence for hydroxysteroid dehydrogenase involvement in the aetiology of

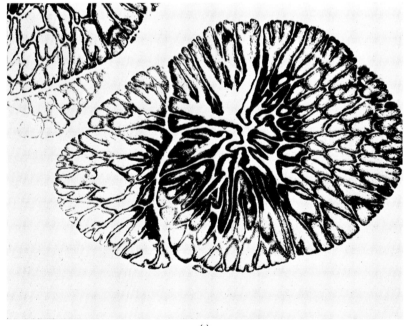

(a)

FIG. 16. (a) a low-power view of the distribution of testosterone-17β-hydroxysteroid dehydrogenase in the avian preen gland. × 30.

acne vulgaris, but we would prefer not to interpret these species differences in this way.

Fish, amphibia and reptiles lack cutaneous sebaceous glands; birds possess a lipid-secreting preen gland which is anatomically and physiologically homologous with the sebaceous glands of mammalian skin. The hydroxy-steroid dehydrogenase activity of this gland appears to be restricted almost entirely to a 17β-hydroxysteroid dehydrogenase; only trace or weak 3α-, 3β-and 16β-hydroxysteroid dehydrogenase activity can be demonstrated. The 17β-hydroxysteroid dehydrogenase activity is particularly intense (Fig. 16) and its substrate specificity is summarized in Table 2. At the present time it seems unwise to speculate on the possible function of the avian preen gland 17β-hydroxysteroid dehydrogenase; the histochemical resemblance of the preen gland to human sebaceous glands is intriguing, however.

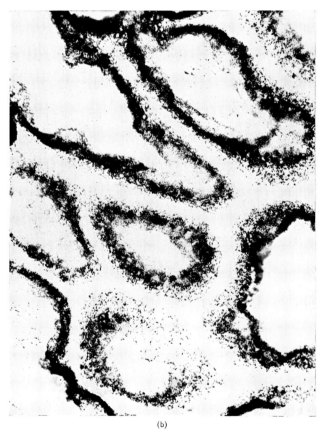

(b)

FIG. 16. Continued. (b) A high-power view of avian preen gland testosterone-17β-hydroxy-steroid dehydrogenase. × 160.

TABLE 2

Substrate specificity of 17β-hydroxysteroid dehydrogenase

Testosterone	+ + +
Oestradiol-17β	+
17β-Hydroxy-5α-androstan-3-one	+
17β-Hydroxy-5β-androstan-3-one	trace
Testosterone propionate	+ +
Testosterone decanoate	+ +
Testosterone isocaproate	+ +
Testosterone phenyl propionate	–

REFERENCES

Baillie, A. H., Calman, K. C. and Milne, J. A. (1965). Histochemical distribution of hydroxysteroid dehydrogenases in human skin. *Brit. J. Dermatol.* **77**, 610–616.

Baillie, A. H., Thomson, J. L. and Milne, J. A. (1966). Anatomical age and sex distribution of hydroxysteroid dehydrogenase containing sebaceous glands in human skin. *Brit. J. Dermatol.* (in press).

Cameron, E. H. D., Baillie, A. H., Grant, J. K., Milne, J. A. and Thomson, J. (1966). Transformation *in vitro* of [7α-^{3}H]dehydroepiandrosterone to [^{3}H]testosterone by skin from men. *J. Endocrinol.* (in press).

Pochi, P. E., Strauss, J. S. and Mescon, H. (1962). Sebum secretion and urinary fractional 17-ketosteroid and total 17-hydroxycorticoid excretion in male castrates. *J. Invest. Dermatol.* **39**, 475–483.

Pochi, P. E., Strauss, J. S. and Mescon, H. (1963). The role of adrenal cortical-steroids in the control of human sebaceous gland activity. *J. Invest. Dermatol.* **41**, 391–399.

Strauss, J. S. and Pochi, P. E. (1963). The Sebaceous glands. *Advances in Biology of Skin*, Vol. 4 Ch. 14. (Pergamon, Oxford and London).

Strauss, J. S., Kligman, A. M. and Pochi, P. E. (1962). The effect of androgens and estrogens on human sebaceous glands. *J. Invest. Dermatol.* **39**, 139–155.

CHAPTER 3

The Genital Ridge and Indifferent Gonad

I. THE GENITAL RIDGE

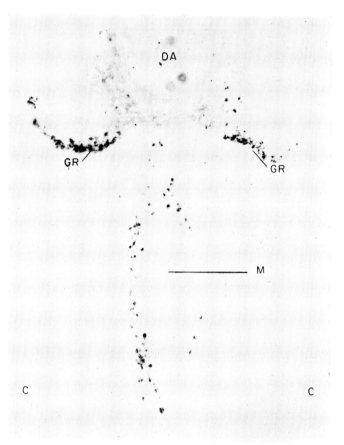

FIG. 17. A transverse section through a 14 mm human embryo showing alkaline phosphatase in the germ cells in the dorsal mesentery (M) of the gut and in the genital ridge (GR) on each side of the root of the dorsal mesentery. The dorsal aorta (DA) and coelomic (C) or peritoneal cavity are also shown. × 60.

The genital ridges (Fig. 17) constitute paired mesenchymal primordia which project, on each side of the dorsal mesentery, from the medial aspect

34

of the mesonephroi. The genital ridge has a mesenchymal core consisting of simple stellate or spindle-shaped cells, whose boundaries are difficult to define, and a covering of rapidly proliferating coelomic epithelium. Large primordial germ or sex cells can be seen migrating into the genital ridge from gut endoderm or its associated mesoderm (Fig. 17); these large and unusual cells can be characterized by their high alkaline phosphatase activity (McKay *et al.*, 1953).

The first histochemical evidence of steroid metabolism was the observation (Hart *et al.*, 1966) of weak NAD-linked 16β-hydroxysteroid dehydrogenase activity in the genital ridge of a very early mouse embryo. In the mesenchyme of the genital ridge of a 14 mm human foetus (Baillie *et al.*, 1966) the presence of 3α-, Δ^5-3β-, 16β- and 17β-hydroxysteroid (Figs. 18 and 19) dehydrogenases,

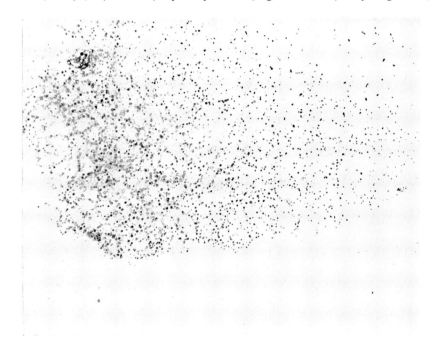

FIG. 18. Δ^5-3β-Hydroxysteroid dehydrogenase activity in the genital ridge of the (14 mm) foetus shown in Fig. 17. DHA was employed as substrate. × 250.

in histochemically demonstrable amounts, have been recorded. These results suggest that conversions 1–6 in Fig. 20 can be undertaken, provided that suitable isomerases and other appropriate enzymes are present.

It will be seen from Fig. 20 that the genital ridge mesenchyme has the theoretical ability to produce a variety of androgens including testosterone, androsterone and androstenedione from DHA. Cholesterol biosynthesis is not yet established biochemically in the genital ridge, but DHA of maternal or placental origin is readily available to the foetus. The possible synthesis of

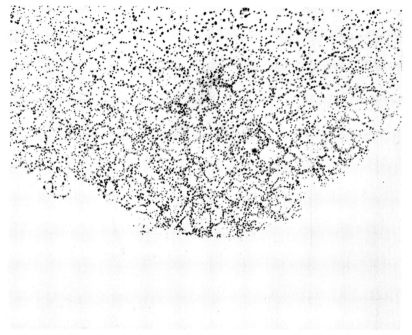

FIG. 19. 17β-Hydroxysteroid dehydrogenase in the genital ridge of a 14 mm human foetus, using oestradiol as substrate. × 250.

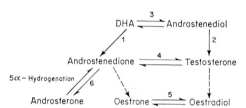

FIG. 20. Reactions 1 and 2 are catalysed by Δ^5-3β-hydroxysteroid dehydrogenase, reactions 3–5 by 17β-hydroxysteroid dehydrogenase and reaction 6 by 3α-hydroxysteroid dehydrogenase.

androgens or oestrogens by the genital ridge mesenchyme is clearly of profound importance in early gonadal embryogenesis, and these histochemical findings raise the possibility that the chemotactic agents believed to control germ cell migration (Woods, 1902; Firket, 1913, 1920; Willier, 1939; Witschi, 1948; Johnston, 1951) are steroidal in nature. On reaching the genital ridge the primitive sex cells undergo extensive and rapid mitosis (Mintz, 1957), and it may be that this mitotic activity, together with that known to occur in the coelomic epithelium at this time is controlled by local concentrations of steroids in the genital ridge.

II. The Indifferent Gonad

The mesenchyme of the indifferent human gonad (Gillman, 1948) adopts a cord-like arrangement as early as the 6·7 mm stage, and the mesenchymal cells, whatever their embryonic origin, progressively adopt a radial arrangement between the developing sex cords. Primordial sex cells are visible in the mesenchyme at this stage. The indifferent gonad enjoys only a very brief existence as such before the onset of sex determination, and most histochemists have not been fortunate enough to include indifferent gonad in their series on developing ovaries or testes.

Only the mouse indifferent gonad has been examined for hydroxysteroid dehydrogenases, and no data are at present available for Man. The mouse testis is first histologically recognizable (Brambell, 1927) on the eleventh day of foetal life, and the intertubular mesenchymal cells do not adopt the appearance of morphologically typical Leydig cells until considerably later (Roosen-Runge and Anderson, 1959). In the mesenchyme of the 11-day foetal mouse gonad, pregnenolone gives a weak 3β-hydroxysteroid dehydrogenase reaction (Baillie and Griffiths, 1964), although other 3β-hydroxysteroids including 17α-hydroxypregnenolone and DHA are not histochemically utilized. These results have been confirmed (Hart et al., 1966) and the presence of a 16β-hydroxysteroid dehydrogenase has also been established in the indifferent gonad mesenchyme. 3α-, 6β-, 11β-, 16α- and 17β-Hydroxysteroids give no histochemical reaction in the interstitium of indifferent mouse gonads.

In the indifferent gonads and interrenal tissue of Pleurodeles waltlii and Xenopus Laevis (Rapola, 1962; Collenot, 1964; Gallien et al., 1964) Δ^5-3β-hydroxysteroid dehydrogenase activity is histochemically demonstrable. These results point to a surprising similarity in early amphibian and mammalian gonadal development and indicate the possibility of steroidogenesis from the moment the gonad is first recognizable.

REFERENCES

Baillie, A. H. and Griffiths, K. (1964). 3β-Hydroxysteroid dehydrogenase activity in the mouse Leydig cell. J. Endocrinol. 29, 9–17.
Baillie, A. H., Ferguson, M. M. and Hart, D. McK. (1966). Evidence of steroid metabolism and possible biosynthesis in the human genital ridge mesenchyme. J. Clin. Endocrinol. 26, 738.
Brambell, F. W. R. (1927). The development and morphology of the gonads of the mouse. I. The morphogenesis of the indifferent gonad and of the ovary Proc. Roy. Soc. (London), Ser. B 101, 391–409.
Collenot, A. (1964). Mise en evidence histochimique d'une Δ^5-3β-hydroxystéroide-déshydrogenase dans les gonades non différenciées et en cours de differenciation des mâles génétiques de l'Urodèle. Compt. Rend. 259, 2535–2537.
Firket, J. (1913). Recherches sur les genocytes, primaires (Urgenchlechtszellen) pendant la periode d'indifférence sexuelle et le developpement de l'ovaire chez le poulet. Anat. Am. 44, 166–175.
Firket, J. (1920). On the origin of germ cells in higher vertebrates. Anat. Record 18, 309–316.

Gallien, L., Certain, P. and Ozon, R. (1964). Mise en evidence d'une Δ^5-3β-hydroxy-steroid deshydrogenase dans le tissue interrenal de l'urodele *Pleurodeles waltlii* Michah aux divers stades du développement. *Compt. Rend.* **258**, 5729–5731.

Gillman, J. (1948). The development of the gonads in man, with a consideration of the role of foetal endocrines and the histogenesis of ovarian tumours. *Contrib. Embryol. Carnegie Inst.* **210**, 81–131.

Hart, D. McK., Baillie, A. H., Calman, K. C. and Ferguson, M. M. (1966). Hydroxy-steroid dehydrogenase development in the mouse adrenal and gonads. *J. Anat. (London)* (in press).

Johnston, P. M. (1951). The embryonic history of the germ cells of the large mouth black bass, *Micropterus salmoides salmoides* (Lacepede). *J. Morphol.* **88**, 471–542.

McKay, D. G., Hertig, A. T., Adams, E. C. and Danziger, S. (1953). Histochemical observations on the germ cells of human embryos. *Anat. Record* **117**, 201–219.

Mintz, B. (1957). Embryological development of primordial germ cells in the mouse. Influence of a new mutation. *J. Embryol. Exptl. Morphol.* **5**, 396–403.

Rapola, J. (1962). Role of hormones in gonadal development. *Ann. Acad. Sci. Fennicae* **64**, 1–81.

Roosen-Runge, E. C. and Anderson, D. (1959). The development of the interstitial cells in the testis of the albino rat. *Acta Anat.* **37**, 125–137.

Willier, B. H. (1939). The embryonic development of sex. In: *Sex and Internal Secretions* (Allen, Ed.) pp. 64–144 (Baillière, Tindall and Cox, London).

Witschi, E. (1948). Migration of the germ cells of human embryos from the yolk-sac to the primitive gonadal folds. *Carnegie Inst. Wash. Publ.* No. 575. *Contrib. Embryol.* **32**, 67–80.

Woods, F. A. (1902). Origin and migration of the germ cells in *acanthias*. *Am. J. Anat.* **1**, 307–320.

CHAPTER 4

The Testis and Epididymis

I. THE LEYDIG TISSUE

A. 3α-HYDROXYSTEROID DEHYDROGENASE

3α-Hydroxysteroid dehydrogenase was first described histochemically in the Leydig cells of adult mouse and human testes by Baillie *et al.* (1966). The reaction is both NAD- and NADP-linked and is not particularly strong (Fig. 21), monoformazan mainly being deposited in the Leydig cells. The seminiferous tubules are difficult to control with this reaction but are probably

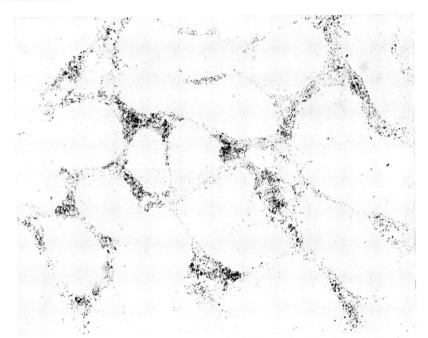

FIG. 21. 3α-hydroxysteroid dehydrogenase activity in human Leydig cells; note the absence of activity in the seminiferous tubules. × 90.

completely negative. In a fairly large series of human testes, Baillie and Mack (1966) record that 3α-hydroxysteroids with either the *cis* or *trans* ring junction give an equally strong reaction in human Leydig cells; in mouse Leydig cells 3α-hydroxysteroids with a 5α-configuration are better utilized than the corresponding 5β-steroids. The biochemical significance of this reaction is outlined in Fig. 22. The existence of a testicular 3α-hydroxysteroid dehydrogenase might have been anticipated by the isolation of naturally occurring 3α-hydroxysteroids from rabbit, guinea-pig and boar testes (Prelog and Ruzicka, 1944; Gower and Haslewood, 1961).

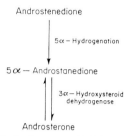

FIG. 22. A biochemical role for 3α-hydroxysteroid dehydrogenase in androgen metabolism.

Goldberg *et al.* (1964) have failed to obtain a colour reaction in human testes incubated with a variety of 3α-hydroxysteroids including androstane and pregnane derivatives. These authors fail to state the delay between excision and freezing of the tissue, and their results are at variance with both biochemical and other histochemical data.

In the mouse trace 3α-hydroxysteroid dehydrogenase is first demonstrable in the testis of the 15 day foetal mouse, and the enzyme is constantly present in the interstitium of the testes of all foetal mice aged 17 days and over (Fig. 23). In the human foetal testis (Hart *et al.*, 1966b) weak 3α-hydroxysteroid

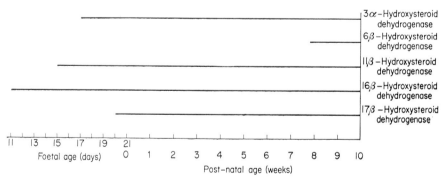

FIG. 23. Histogram of the age of appearance of different hydroxysteroid dehydrogenases in the developing mouse testis.

dehydrogenase activity is present in the testis of a 4·3 cm embryo and in all older gonads surveyed. The volume of Leydig tissue in the postnatal mouse capable of undertaking 3α-dehydrogenation has been established (Hart *et al.*, 1966a) and shows a regular increase with age (Fig. 24),

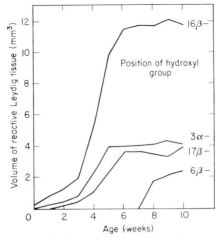

Fig. 24. The volume of Leydig tissue having different hydroxysteroid dehydrogenases changes with age and increases as the animal (mouse) approaches maturity.

B. Δ^5-3β-HYDROXYSTEROID DEHYDROGENASE

This was first demonstrated biochemically by Samuels *et al.* (1951) and is a cardinal enzyme in steroid biosynthesis. Its role is indicated in Fig. 10.

A substantial amount of biochemical work points to its existence in human, stallion (Savard and Goldzieher, 1960; Engel and Langer, 1961), dog (Brinck-Johnsen and Eik-Nes, 1957; Aakvaag *et al.*, 1964; Hagen and Eik-Nes, 1964), pig (Koch, 1944; Neher and Wettstein, 1960), guinea-pig (Gower and Haslewood, 1961), rabbit (Rosner *et al.*, 1964), rat (Savard and Dorfman, 1954; Samuels and Helmreich, 1956; Mosebach *et al.*, 1963) testes, but at the present time it is uncertain whether this is a single enzyme, or a number of closely related enzymes, as the corresponding Δ^5–Δ^4 isomerases appear to be (Ewald *et al.*, 1964; Kruskemper *et al.*, 1964).

Wattenberg, in 1958, was the first to localize 3β-hydroxysteroid dehydrogenase in the interstitial cells of the rabbit testis using pregnenolone and DHA as substrates. Testicular 3β-hydroxysteroid dehydrogenase has subsequently been explored in three principal ways. First, several workers have deliberately looked for alternative 3β-hydroxysteroid substrates; secondly, the species distribution of testicular 3β-hydroxysteroid dehydrogenase has been explored; and finally the development of this enzyme or enzymes with age has been studied in the testes of various species. Most histochemists have accepted the statement of Beyer and Samuels (1956) that NAD was the required co-enzyme, and to date investigators have not sought an NADP-dependent 3β-hydroxysteroid dehydrogenase in the testis histochemically.

The *substrate-specificity* of testicular 3β-hydroxysteroid dehydrogenase was rapidly explored in the testis. Wattenberg (1958) first used pregnenolone and

DHA, and these have remained the standard substrates. Hitzeman (1962) extended this range to include the 17α-methyl derivative of androstenediol, a configuration which is now known to impair the oxidation of the 17β-hydroxyl group. Baillie and Griffiths (1964) noted that 17α-hydroxypregnenolone served as a satisfactory substrate in murine Leydig cells, but the reaction was weaker than that observed with pregnenolone and DHA. The fourth physiological substrate (Fig. 25), androstenediol, was shown to give a good colour reaction in murine Leydig cells in 1965, but a part of this colour reaction at least is probably due to oxidation of the 17β-hydroxyl function. In the same year (Baillie, 1965; Baillie and Griffiths, 1965b) pregnenediol and 16α-hydroxypregnenolone were shown to be utilized histochemically by murine Leydig cells (Fig. 25), although the corresponding 3-keto 16α- or 20β-hydroxy-

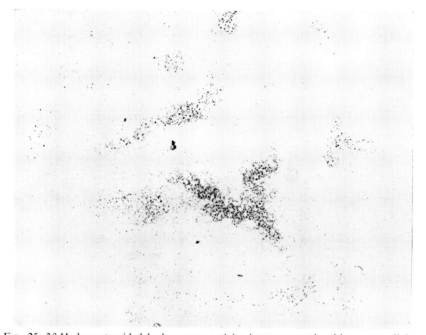

FIG. 25. 3β-Hydroxysteroid dehydrogenase activity in mouse testis with pregnenediol as substrate: activity is confined to the Leydig cells. × 200.

steroids gave no colour. Cholesterol, lanosterol, 3β-hydroxyandrost-5,16-dien-17-one, 3β-hydroxy-5β-androstan, 3β-hydroxy-5β-androstan-17-one and 3β,17β-dihydroxy-5β-androstan have all been used as substrates in the histochemical demonstration of Δ⁵-3β- and 3β-hydroxysteroid dehydrogenase (A. H. Baillie, unpublished observations) in the testis. Saturated steroids with the 5β-configuration and Δ⁵ steroids give a good colour, but the reaction is influenced by the 17-configuration. 17-Keto- or 17β-hydroxysteroids give an intense reaction, but the use of 17β-hydroxysteroids is, in general terms, to be avoided in view of the alternative hydrogen source in the molecule.

Pathways alternative to the well-established one involving pregnenolone–progesterone–17α-hydroxyprogesterone–androstenedione have been postulated by Engel and Langer (1961). Similar alternative pathways are now well established in adrenal tissue by various workers (Goldstein *et al.*, 1960; Lipsett and Hökfelt, 1961; Mulrow *et al.*, 1962; Weliky and Engel, 1962, 1963). These pathways are detailed in Fig. 10, and from the histochemical data available in the testis the conversions DHA–androstenedione and androstenediol-testosterone appear to be much greater than conversions 1 and 2 in Fig. 10. Whether or not this is a function of 17-substitution is unclear. It would certainly seem that removal of the cholesterol or pregnenolone side-chain facilitates 3β-dehydrogenation, at least histochemically.

Of more contemporary interest, however, are the histochemical results obtained with the 3β-sulphoxysteroids. Although the precise metabolic role of the steroid sulphates in steroid hormone biosynthesis remains unknown, several reports on metabolism of steroid sulphates have appeared in the literature. In the mouse testis (Baillie and Griffiths, 1965b) pregnenolone sulphate and 17α-hydroxypregnenolone sulphate gave histochemical colour reactions in the Leydig cells. DHA sulphate gave a weak reaction only in the seminiferous epithelium (Fig. 26). This reaction coincided with the development of mature spermatozoa in the tubules both temporally and histologically. Although the precise role of DHA sulphate is unclear, the possibility that the seminiferous epithelium constitutes a target organ for this steroid should not

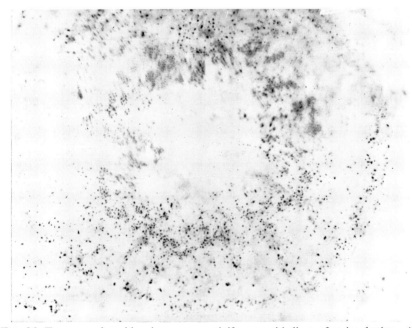

FIG. 26. Formazan deposition in mouse seminiferous epithelium after incubation with DHA sulphate. × 350.

be dismissed. It gives a reaction (A. H. Baillie, unpublished) in ovine semi-niferous tubules.

In the human foetal testis the 3β-sulphoxy derivatives of pregnenolone and 17α-hydroxypregnenolone give a histochemical reaction in the Leydig cells of foetuses longer than 3·0 cm (Baillie *et al.*, 1965a). In pubertal and adult human testes (Baillie and Mack, 1966) a strong histochemical reaction (Fig. 27) occurs in the Leydig cells of almost all human testes with pregnenolone

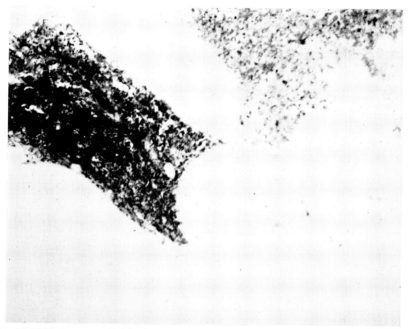

FIG. 27. 3β-Hydroxysteroid dehydrogenase activity in the interstitium of an abnormal human testis after incubation with DHA sulphate. To date we have seen three such testes charac-terized by arrest of spermatid maturation and increased activity of hydroxysteroid de-hydrogenases in the Leydig cells. × 140.

sulphate, 17α-hydroxypregnenolone sulphate and DHA sulphate. The reaction with the 3β-sulphoxy steroids is particularly intense in the Leydig cells of cryptorchid testes. The sulphates were also used by a testis from a chromatin-positive example of Klinefelter's syndrome. The mechanism of the colour reaction involved in the histochemical utilization of steroid sulphates is unclear; the most likely explanation seems to be that the sulphoxy derivatives are converted to the free steroid, which then undergoes dehydro-genation, but proof for this supposition is lacking.

Exploration of the *species distribution* of testicular Δ⁵-3β-hydroxysteroid dehydrogenase has only commenced relatively recently, and the results are summarized in Table 3. Reference to Table 3 indicates, at least in the primates, some conflict of results, and there are two clearly opposed groups of workers.

Deane and Rubin (1965) and Maeir (1965), on the one hand, report that Δ^5-3β-hydroxysteroid dehydrogenase is not histochemically demonstrable in human Leydig cells; Goldberg *et al.* (1963), in a fairly large series of normal human testes, record similar negative results, except in one testis which had demonstrable Δ^5-3β-hydroxysteroid dehydrogenase activity. Moreover, Goldberg *et al.* (1964) state that DHA is not used by human testes. On the other hand, Baillie *et al.* (1965) and Baillie and Mack (1966) have described Δ^5-3β-hydroxy-

TABLE 3

Species distribution of Leydig cell Δ^5-3β-hydroxysteroid dehydrogenase

Class	Animal	Present	Substrates and comments	Investigator
Pisces	Gobius pagannellus	Yes	Pregnenolone and DHA. The reaction is weakest at the beginning of a new annual cycle	Stanley et al. (1965)
	Tilapia Mossambica	Yes	Pregnenolone and DHA	Yaron (1966)
	Torpedo marmorata	Yes	DHA	Della Corte et al. (1961)
	Scyliorhinus stellaris Selachii	Yes	Present in Leydig cells	Chieffi et al. (1963)
	Morone lubrax	Yes	DHA	Lupo and Chieffi (1963)
	Selachii	Yes	DHA	Collenot and Ozon (1964)
Amphibia	Triton cristatus	Yes	Pregnenolone, 17α-hydroxy-pregnenolone, DHA and androstenediol	A. H. Baillie (unpublished)
	Triturus cristatus	Yes	DHA	Della Corte et al. (1962)
	Rana esculenta	Yes	DHA	Chieffi and Botte (1963)
	Pleurodeles waltlii	Yes	DHA	Certain et al. (1964)
Reptilia	Chrysemis sp. Varanus niloticus L. Natrix natrix L.	Yes	DHA	Arvy (1962)
		Yes	DHA	Botte (1963)
Aves	Gallus domesticus	Yes	Pregnenolone, 17α-hydroxypregnenolone, DHA and androstenediol	A. H. Baillie (unpublished)
	Gallus gallus Perdix perdix Coturnix coturnix Phasianus colchicus L. Alectoris rufa L.	Yes	DHA	Arvy (1962)
	Gallus domesticus	Yes	DHA	Chieffi (1964)
	Gallus domesticus	Yes	DHA	Narbaitz and Kolodny (1964)
Mammalia	Didelphys virginiana Metachirus nudicaudatus	Yes	DHA-activity in the seminiferous epithelium as well as the Leydig cells	Maeir (1965)
	Rattus rattus and R. norvegicus	(a) Yes	Pregnenolone and DHA	Pearson and Grose (1959a)
		(b) Yes	DHA	Arvy (1962)
		(c) Yes	Pregnenolone and DHA	Niemi and Ikonen, (1962)
		(d) Yes	DHA	Fuhrmann (1963)
		(e) Yes	Pregnenolone 17α-hydroxypregnenolone DHA	Goldman et al. (1965)
		(f) Yes	DHA	Maeir (1965)
	Cavia porcellus (guinea-pig)	(a) Yes	DHA	Price et al. (1964)
		(b) Yes	DHA	Maeir (1965)
		(c) Yes	Pregnenolone, 17α-hydroxypregnenolone, DHA and androstenediol	A. H. Baillie (unpublished)
	Mus musculus (mouse)	(a) Yes	Pregnenolone, DHA, 17α-methyl androstenediol	Hitzeman (1962)
		(b) Yes	DHA	Cavallero et al. (1963)
		(c) Yes	Pregnenolone 17α-hydroxypregnenolone DHA	Baillie and Griffiths (1965 a, b)
		(d) Yes	DHA	Magrini and Martinazzi (1964)

TABLE 3. Continued

Class	Animal	Present	Substrates and comments	Investigator
		(e) Yes	16α-Hydroxypregnenolone, pregnenediol, androstenediol, pregnenolone sulphate, 17α-hydroxypregnenolone sulphate, DHA sulphate	Baillie and Griffiths (1965); Baillie (1965)
		(f) Yes	DHA	Maeir (1965)
	Mesocricetus auratus (hamster)	(a) Yes	DHA	Maeir (1965)
		(b) Yes	Pregnenolone, 17α-hydroxypregnenolone, DHA	A. H. Baillie (unpublished)
	Oryctolagus cuniculus (rabbit)	(a) Yes	Pregnenolone, DHA	Wattenberg (1958)
		(b) Yes	DHA	Maeir (1965)
	Myotis lucifugus (bat)	Yes	DHA	Maeir (1965)
	Canis familiaris (dog)	(a) Yes	DHA	Maeir (1965)
		(b) Yes	Pregnenolone, 17α-hydroxypregnenolone, androstenediol	A. H. Baillie (unpublished)
	Felis catus (cat)	(a) Yes	DHA	Maeir (1965)
	Mephitis mephitis nigra (skunk)	Yes	DHA	Maeir (1965)
	Macaca mulatta (rhesus monkey)	(a) No	Pregnenolone, DHA and their sulphates	Maeir (1965)
		(b) Yes	Pregnenolone, 17α-hydroxypregnenolone, DHA and their sulphates	A. H. Baillie (unpublished)
	Homo sapiens (man)	(a) Yes	Pregnenolone and DHA	Jirasek and Raboch (1963)
		(b) Yes	Pregnenolone and DHA	Mancini et al. (1963)
		(c) Yes	Foetal ⎰Pregnenolone, 17α-hydroxypregnenolone DHA and their sulphates⎱	Baillie et al. (1965a)
		(d) Yes	Adult	Baillie and Mack (1966)
		(e) No	Pregnenolone and DHA	Goldberg et al. (1963)
		(f) No	Androstenediol, 3β, 17α-dihydroxyandrost-5-ene pregnenolone, pregnanediol	Goldberg et al. (1964)
		(g) Yes	Androstenediol, DHA, epiandrosterone, pregnenediol, androstenediol dipropionate	Goldberg et al. (1964)
		(h) No	Pregnenolone, DHA and their sulphates	Maeir (1965) Deane and Rubin (1965)
		(i) No	Not known	Quoted by Maier (1965)
		(j) Yes	DHA-foetal testes react from the point of sex differentiation	Cavallero et al. (1965)
		(k) Yes	DHA-foetal testes	Magrini (1965)
		(l) Yes	Pregnenolone and DHA neonatal testes	Goldman et al. (1966)

steroid dehydrogenase activity in foetal, pre-pubertal and adult human testes with a variety of substrates; similar findings have been reported independently in other laboratories (Jirasek and Raboch, 1963; Mancini et al., 1963). It should be clearly noted that Baillie and Mack (1966) studied almost 50 human testes and that the age and substrate range investigated was very wide.

It is difficult to reconcile these widely divergent views, but the following points give an indication of the possibilities. First, the Goldberg et al. (1964) paper is equivocal in that these workers note Δ^5-3β-hydroxysteroid dehydrogenase in human Leydig cells with some steroids but not with others. Secondly, we have noted that washing of the sections in buffer or acetone prior to incubation reduces or abolishes demonstrable Δ^5-3β-hydroxysteroid dehydrogenase activity. Those workers who fail to detect 3β-hydroxysteroid dehydrogenase activity in the human testis invariably wash their sections, and in our experience the enzyme is readily demonstrable in human Leydig cells, provided that preliminary washing is avoided; this accords with most of the bio-chemical evidence (Dorfman *et al.*, 1963).

Age changes in the distribution of testicular Δ⁵-3β-hydroxysteroid dehydro-genase have been most extensively studied by Baillie (1965) and Baillie and Griffiths (1965a, b). In the foetus, murine Leydig cells acquire the ability to dehydrogenate different 3β-substrates at different ages (Fig. 28) and the path-

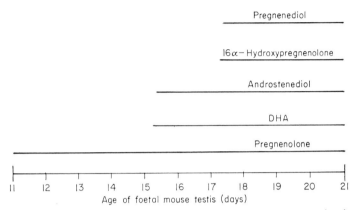

FIG. 28. Age at which 3β-hydroxy substrates first give a histochemical reaction in murine Leydig cells.

way involving the conversion of pregnenolone to progesterone is the first to appear histochemically. In the foetal human Leydig cells the progressive development (Baillie *et al.*, 1965a) of histochemical utilization of various 3β-hydroxysteroids resembles that seen in the mouse.

In the post-natal mouse testis (Baillie and Griffiths, 1964, 1965b) the volume of Leydig tissue capable of histochemically utilizing the various 3β-hydroxy-steroids changes with age. The volume of tissue capable of acting on pregneno-lone and related steroids is represented in Fig. 29. It will be seen that after birth it rises initially with age (Fig. 29) and falls with the approach of adult life. 17α-Hydroxypregnenolone (Fig. 30) is not utilized till late in post-natal life, and the volume of tissue metabolizing this steroid behaves quite differently from the volume of tissue which metabolizes pregnenolone.

DHA and androstenediol are both well utilized by the post-natal mouse interstitium (Figs. 31 and 32), and the growth curves of reactive tissue are sigmoid in form. Of the two, androstenediol is much better utilized histo-chemically (Figs. 31 and 32), but the possibility of 17β-dehydrogenation contributing to formazan deposition with this steroid cannot be excluded.

The different times of onset of foetal utilization of the various substrates, considered together with the differing metabolic activities of the post-natal interstitium, can most conveniently be explained by postulating the existence of different, substrate-specific Δ⁵-3β-hydroxysteroid dehydrogenases. Baillie and Mack (1966) described two abnormal human testes which exhibited normal

Δ^5-3β-hydroxysteroid dehydrogenase when incubated with pregnenolone, 17α-hydroxypregnenolone or androstenediol, but which failed entirely to utilize DHA. This observation (see Fig. 10) could readily be explained by the absence of a specific DHA-3β-hydroxysteroid dehydrogenase. It is interesting to note in this connection that the corresponding Δ^5-3-oxosteroid isomerases have been shown to be highly substrate-specific (Ewald *et al.*, 1964; Kruskemper *et al.*, 1964). Although in our view substrate-specific 3β-hydroxysteroid dehydrogenases are the most likely explanation of the testicular histochemical results, it is possible that the substrate specific isomerases in some

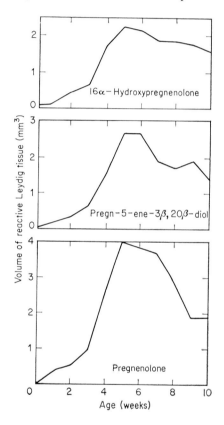

FIG. 29. Age changes in the volume of murine Leydig tissue capable of dehydrogenating several 3β-hydroxysteroids. Compare with Figs. 31–33. (From Baillie and Griffiths, 1965: reproduced by courtesy of *J. Endocrinol.*).

way influence 3β-dehydrogenation. Solubility factors and membrane permeability effects cannot be wholly excluded but seem to us unlikely explanations.

The key role of Δ^5-3β-hydroxysteroid dehydrogenase in steroid biosynthesis has been noted (see Fig. 10) and the histochemical findings point to the bulk

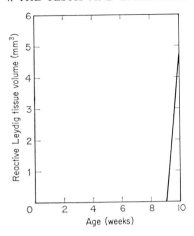

FIG. 30. 3β-Hydroxysteroid dehydrogenase in murine Leydig cells only dehydrogenates 17α-hydroxypregnenolone as adult life approaches. (From Baillie and Griffiths, 1964: reproduced by courtesy of *J. Endocrinol.*).

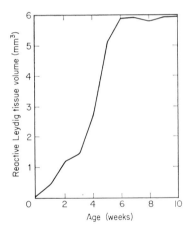

FIG. 31. The volume of murine Leydig tissue capable of dehydrogenating DHA increases regularly with age. (From Baillie and Griffiths, 1964: reproduced by courstesy of *J. Endocrinol.*).

of such biosynthesis as being located in the intertubular cells of Leydig. Nevertheless, Maeir (1965) has drawn attention to a 3β-hydroxysteroid dehydrogenase in marsupial seminiferous tubules, and in human tubules persistent trace 3β-hydroxysteroid dehydrogenase activity is encountered. These facts are more fully discussed in Section II of this chapter.

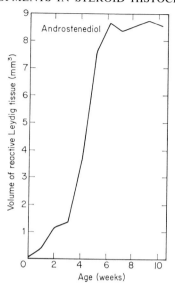

F IG. 32. The volume of Leydig tissue in the mouse testis capable of metabolizing andro-stenediol exhibits a sigmoid growth curve with age. Maximal growth occurs in the third and fourth weeks of post-natal life. (From Baillie and Griffiths, 1965: reproduced by courtesy of *J. Endocrinol.*)

C. 6β-HYDROXYSTEROID DEHYDROGENASE

In a preliminary paper (Baillie *et al.*, 1966) some evidence of weak 6β-hydroxysteroid dehydrogenase activity was noted in the Leydig cells of mouse and some human testes. The reaction was weak and NAD-linked. Hart *et al.* (1966a) have established that 6β-hydroxysteroid dehydrogenase activity occurs in the Leydig cells of adult albino mice but is absent from murine Leydig cells before the end of the eighth week of post-natal life. In ten out of fifteen normal adult human testes examined (Baillie and Mack, 1966) weak 6β-hydroxysteroid dehydrogenase was observed in the Leydig cells. In both species, however, the reaction is inconstant and unconvincing. 6β-Hydroxy-steroids occur naturally as cortisol (Ulstrom *et al.*, 1960) or oestrogen (Breuer *et al.*, 1958) derivatives.

D. 11β-HYDROXYSTEROID DEHYDROGENASE

11β-Hydroxysteroid dehydrogenase activity was first described histo-chemically in human and murine Leydig cells by Baillie *et al.*, 1965c. The enzyme utilizes either NAD or NADP in the testis and its substrate preference is indicated in Table 4. From Table 4 it is clear that 11β-hydroxyandro-stenedione and 11β-hydroxyprogesterone are the substrates of choice. In human interstitial cells (Fig. 33) a moderate 11β-hydroxysteroid dehydrogenase is apparent consistently (Baillie and Mack, 1966). In murine testis (Fig. 34)

TABLE 4

11β-Hydroxysteroid dehydrogenase activity of human
Leydig tissue incubated with various substrates

Substrate	Reactive Leydig tissue (%)
Androstenedione	—
11β-Hydroxyandrostenedione	4·5
Oestrone	—
11β-Hydroxyoestrone	1·8
Progesterone	—
11β-Hydroxyprogesterone	4·4

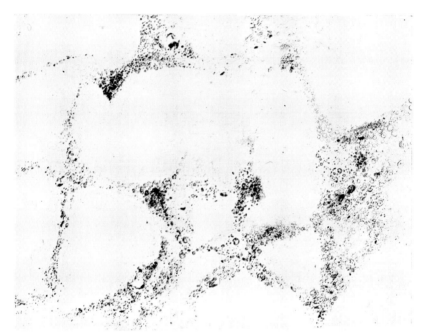

FIG. 33. 11β-Hydroxysteroid dehydrogenase activity in human Leydig tissue with 11β-hydroxyandrostenedione as substrate. × 130.

the volume of Leydig tissue with 11β-hydroxysteroid dehydrogenase activity increases regularly with age.

Of more importance, from the point of view of testicular endocrine function, is the fact that 11β-hydroxysteroid dehydrogenase may interconvert a number of 11β-hydroxy and 11-keto androgens (Fig. 35). Biochemically an 11β-hydroxylase and an 11β-hydroxysteroid dehydrogenase are known to exist in normal and abnormal testicular material (Savard et al., 1960; Smith *et al.*, 1964) and the conversions proposed in Fig. 15 can be ascribed to the Leydig cells. The production of 11β-hydroxyandrostenedione, 11β-hydroxyandrosterone, 11β-hydroxytestosterone and 11β-hydroxyaetiocholanolone, together with their corresponding 11-keto derivatives, is now well established in human (Savard *et al.*, 1960; Smith *et al.*, 1964) and guinea-pig testes (Hofmann, 1962); the stallion testis (Savard and Goldzieher, 1960) apparently does not have this pathway. 11-Hydroxysteroids of the above type appear to be virilizing, but their biochemical role is uncertain as yet. Amphibian testes lack this enzyme histochemically. (A. H. Baillie, unpublished).

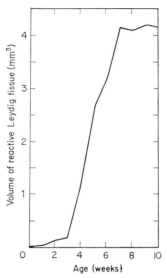

FIG. 34. The sigmoid growth curve of murine Leydig tissue having 11β-hydroxysteroid dehydrogenase activity. (From Baillie *et al.*, 1965: reproduced by courtesy of *J. Endocrinol.*).

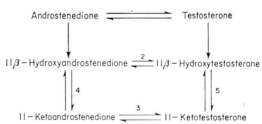

FIG. 35. Reactions 1–3 are catalysed by 17β-hydroxysteroid dehydrogenase; reactions 4 and 5 are carried out by 11β-hydroxysteroid dehydrogenase.

E. 12α-HYDROXYSTEROID DEHYDROGENASE

Baillie *et al.* (1966), in a preliminary paper, reported some evidence of 12α-hydroxysteroid dehydrogenase activity in the Leydig cells of human testes. From further intensive research (Baillie and Mack, 1966) it became clear that 12α-hydroxysteroids were not usually utilized histochemically by human Leydig cells. Murine Leydig cells (Baillie *et al.*, 1966; Hart *et al.*, 1966a) do not utilize 12α-hydroxysteroids to any extent.

F. 16α-HYDROXYSTEROID DEHYDROGENASE

This enzyme is not convincingly present in human or rodent testicular tissue (Baillie *et al.*, 1966; Baillie and Mack, 1966).

G. 16β-HYDROXYSTEROID DEHYDROGENASE

From a histochemical standpoint this enzyme is the most active hydroxy-steroid dehydrogenase in testicular material. The colour reaction is mainly NAD-mediated. The reaction is intense (Fig. 36) and large amounts of di-

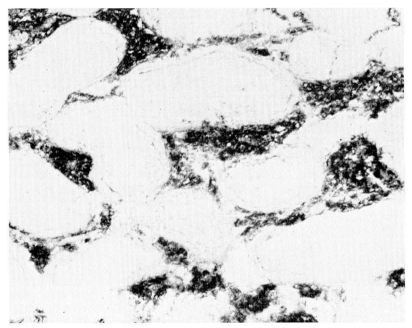

Fig. 36. Intense 16β-hydroxysteroid dehydrogenase activity in human Leydig cells after incubation with 3β,16β-dihydroxyandrost-5-ene 3-methyl ether. (From Baillie and Mack, 1966: reproduced by courtesy of *J. Endocrinol.*). × 130.

formazan are deposited in the Leydig cells. The enzyme occurs in foetal (Hart *et al.*, 1966b) and adult human (Baillie *et al.*, 1966; Baillie and Mack, 1966) Leydig cells, in murine Leydig cells (Baillie *et al.*, 1966), and also in all amphibian, reptilian, avian and mammalian Leydig cells so far studied. Mammalian testes surveyed in this laboratory include cat, dog, rat, guinea-pig, hamster and monkey. Sheep testes are exceptional in that they exhibit poor 16β-hydroxysteroid dehydrogenase activity (A. H. Baillie, unpublished). Seasonal variations have not yet been excluded, however.

In an earlier chapter the presence of 16β-hydroxysteroid dehydrogenase in human and mouse genital ridge was noted. Its presence throughout foetal life in the testicular (Fig. 23) interstitium has been recorded in the mouse (Hart *et al.*, 1966a), and the post-natal growth in volume of intertubular tissue with an active 16β-hydroxysteroid dehydrogenase in that animal is represented in Fig. 24. With regard to substrate-specificity of 16β-hydroxysteroid dehydrogenase in a histochemical system, it has been noted that 16β-hydroxysteroids with an aromatic A-ring are less well used than Δ^4-3-keto steroids.

A bacterial 16β-hydroxysteroid dehydrogenase has been described (Talalay, 1965) but the situation in mammalian tissues is much less well understood. 16α- and 16β-Hydroxysteroids occur in mammalian tissues mostly as oestrogen derivatives (Levitz *et al.*, 1958; Breuer and Nocke, 1959) and the significance of this with respect to testicular metabolism is unclear. Moreover, testicular 16β-hydroxysteroid dehydrogenase appears to prefer 16β-androgens as histochemical substrates, but it would be unwise to infer from this observation that such steroids are its physiological substrates. It is of interest to note that the presence of a 17β-hydroxyl group completely interferes with the histochemical utilization of a 16β-hydroxyl group on the steroid molecule, and this seems to be an example of steric hindrance.

H. 17β-HYDROXYSTEROID DEHYDROGENASE

Histochemical studies of 17β-hydroxysteroid dehydrogenase appear not to have been undertaken following the assertion of Pearson and Grose (1959b) that this enzyme was not histochemically demonstrable in the testis. Hart *et al.* (1966a) have shown that the enzyme appears shortly before birth (Fig. 23) in the mouse testis, and the increase in the volume of Leydig tissue in the postnatal mouse testis capable of undertaking this dehydrogenation is shown in Fig. 24. The enzyme is consistently present in human Leydig cells, and the reaction is NAD- or NADP-linked (Baillie and Mack, 1966). A 17β-hydroxysteroid dehydrogenase (Fig. 38) is also present in the Leydig cells of other species studied in this laboratory, including newts, cockerels, cats, dogs and monkeys.

Goldman *et al.* (1966) found no 17β-hydroxysteroid dehydrogenase in human foetal Leydig cells; one of the writers (A. H. Baillie, unpublished work) has noted activity in several foetal testes. It is interesting to note that Goldberg *et al.* (1964) record a colour with two 17β-hydroxysteroids, androstenediol and the corresponding Δ^5-dipropionate, in human Leydig cells although these workers do not consider the possibility that a 17β-hydroxysteroid dehydrogenase might contribute to their results and attribute the entire colour reaction to a 3β-hydroxysteroid dehydrogenase. The results of Baillie and Mack (1966) make it quite clear that this interpretation is untenable in that human Leydig cells possess histochemically demonstrable 17β-hydroxysteroid dehydrogenase.

From a biochemical standpoint, 17β-hydroxysteroid dehydrogenase carries out the appropriate conversions shown in Fig. 10 and in Fig. 15, Chapter 1; in addition it can catalyse the interconversion of oestrogens such as oestradiol and oestrone. Histochemically, in human and murine Leydig cells no obvious substrate preference exists, and it is therefore possible that any or all of the known interconversions are conducted by the 17β-hydroxysteroid dehydrogenase in these cells.

Fig. 37. 17β-Hydroxysteroid dehydrogenase in the interstitium of the cockerel testis, using testosterone as substrate.

I. 20α-HYDROXYSTEROID DEHYDROGENASE

This enzyme has been shown to exist biochemically (Shikita and Tamaoki, 1965) in human testicular tissue. It is selectively localized in the Leydig cell (Fig. 39) of the human testis (A. H. Baillie, unpublished work), but its physiological role has not been elucidated. It is mainly NADP-linked.

J. 20β-HYDROXYSTEROID DEHYDROGENASE

A very poor histochemical reaction was noted in rodent testis with 20β-hydroxysteroids. In the human testis (Baillie et al., 1965b; Baillie and Mack, 1966) a reasonably strong 20β-hydroxysteroid dehydrogenase is constantly demonstrable (Fig. 39) in the Leydig cells. The reaction is NAD linked. Using 3β, 20β-dihydroxypregn-4-ene, Goldberg et al. (1964) also record a colour

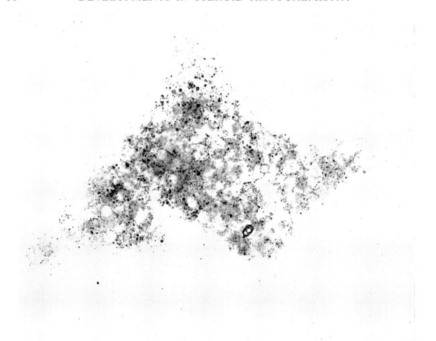

FIG. 38. NADP-linked 20α-hydroxysteroid dehydrogenase in human Leydig cells from an adult testis. × 350.

reaction in human Leydig cells, but these workers have given no consideration to 20β-hydroxysteroid dehydrogenase as a possible hydrogen source and have not controlled the reaction with the appropriate Δ^4-3-keto 20β-hydroxysteroid. 20β-Hydroxysteroid dehydrogenase was first isolated from bacterial sources (Hubener et al., 1959; Hubener and Sahrholtz, 1960); and although human tissues contain both the 20α- and 20β-epimers (Zander et al., 1960), rodent tissues seem to lack the 20β-epimer (Engel and Langer, 1961). These facts would explain the distribution of 20α- and 20β-hydroxysteroid dehydrogenases observed histochemically. It is of interest to note that Acevedo et al. (1963) have established biochemically a 20β-hydroxysteroid dehydrogenase in human foetal testes.

1α-, 1β-, 11α-, 16α- and 17α-Hydroxysteroids consistently give no histochemical reaction in any Leydig tissue (A. H. Baillie, unpublished). 21- and 24-Hydroxysteroids give weak and inconstant reactions in human Leydig tissue (Baillie and Mack, 1966).

K. SUMMARY

In conclusion, the Leydig cells possess a wide variety of hydroxysteroid dehydrogenases including particularly 3α-, 3β-, 11β-, 16β-, 17β- and

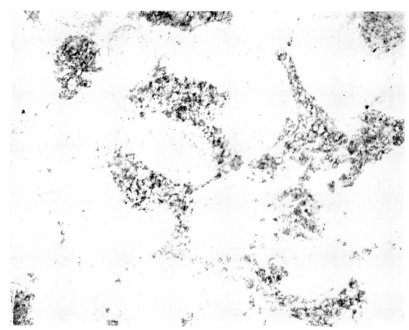

Fig. 39. NAD-linked 20β-hydroxysteroid dehydrogenase in adult human Leydig cells. × 150.

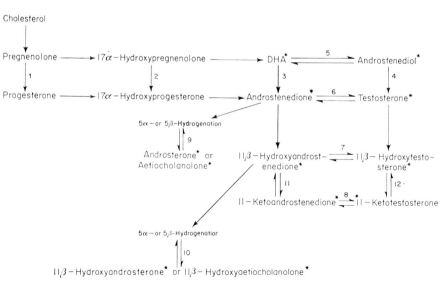

Fig. 40. Reactions 1–4 are due to 3β-hydroxysteroid dehydrogenase. Reactions 5–8 are due
to 17β-hydroxysteroid dehydrogenase. Reactions 9 and 10 are due to 3α-hydroxysteroid
dehydrogenase. Reactions 11 and 12 are due to 11β-hydroxysteroid dehydrogenase. Reactions
1–12 occur in Leydig cells. Asterisks show steroids known to be produced in the testis.

c

20β-hydroxysteroid dehydrogenases. Most of these enzymes can be fitted into a broad biochemical pattern (Fig. 40), but several have not been satisfactorily integrated. Perusal of Fig. 40 suggests that most of the steroids secreted by the testis are produced in the Leydig tissue, when one considers the histochemical results; it must be clearly pointed out, however, that the precise histological location of other enzymes involved in steroidogenesis, including the hydroxylases and sidechain splitting enzymes, is not yet known.

II. The Seminiferous Tubules

Maeir (1965) has recorded substantial Δ^5-3β-hydroxysteroid dehydrogenase activity in marsupial seminiferous tubules, using DHA as substrate. DHA sulphate utilization by mouse seminiferous tubules (Baillie and Griffiths, 1965) has also been observed. Using a variety of substrates, Baillie and Mack (1966) recorded persistent trace Δ^5-3β-hydroxysteroid dehydrogenase in human seminiferous tubules; the extent of the activity is difficult to assess, owing to the difficulty in securing completely colourless controls in human seminiferous tubules, but weak Δ^5-3β-hydroxysteroid dehydrogenase is consistently present in the seminiferous epithelium. In one or two abnormal human testes fairly strong 3β-hydroxysteroid dehydrogenase activity was observable in the tubules.

Baillie and Mack (1966) record quite strong 16β- (Fig. 41) and 17β-hydroxy-

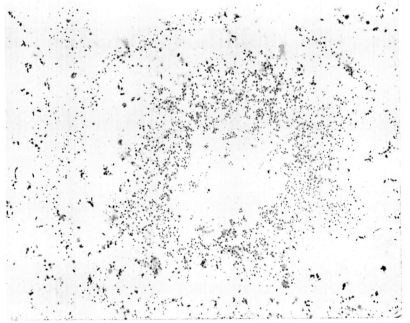

Fig. 41. 16β-Hydroxysteroid dehydrogenase activity in human seminiferous epithelium
× 350.

steroid dehydrogenase activity in all human seminiferous tubules from puberty onwards. In fresh frozen preparations of the type used in hydroxysteroid dehydrogenase histochemistry it is not possible to be sure whether the colour reaction in the Sertoli cells or in the germ cells. Notwithstanding this difficulty, there is clear-cut histochemical evidence for steroid metabolism, and possibly biosynthesis, in the seminiferous tubules.

The occurrence of steroid metabolism in the seminiferous tubules is becoming better documented biochemically. The testis produces oestrogens (Cole et al., 1933; Berthong et al., 1949); it seems that the Sertoli cells may be the principal source of testicular oestrogens (Huggins and Moulder, 1945; Treves, 1958; Griffiths and Grant, 1962). Avian seminiferous tubules contain various progesterones (Lofts and Marshall, 1959) and rat seminiferous tissue has recently been shown to be capable of converting progesterone to 17α-hydroxyprogesterone, androstenedione and testosterone (Christensen and Mason, 1965). The observed 3α-, 16β- and 17β-hydroxysteroid dehydrogenases in primate seminiferous tubules could subserve either oestrogen or androgen metabolism, and at the present time it would be unwise to speculate further on their function.

III. The Rete Testis

The rete testis itself exhibits no evidence of hydroxysteroid dehydrogenase activity.

According to Gillman (1948), the interstitial cells in general give way abruptly in the region where the straight tubules merge with the rete testis, with the result that large interstitial cells are sharply replaced at the boundary of the mediastinum by small stellate or spindle-shaped mesenchymal cells. Leeson (1962) states that the connective tissue surrounding the rat rete is unremarkable from an ultrastructural point of view. A large interstitial cell is infrequently encountered associated with the anastomosing rete tubules.

The connective tissue surrounding the rete testis of the mouse (Baillie, 1961) appears to consist of ordinary fibrous tissue, but a number of enzymes concerned in steroidogenesis and metabolism, including 3α-, 3β- (Fig. 42), 16β- and 17β-hydroxysteroid dehydrogenases are histochemically present in this tissue. In short, the connective tissue of the mediastinal rudiment in the mouse is histochemically undistinguishable from the ordinary Leydig tissue, and presumably produces similar steroids. No evidence regarding the human mediastinum is yet available.

Hooker (1948) has given a detailed description of the cytology of the adult Leydig cells, with particular reference to nuclear structure. Roosen-Runge and Anderson (1959) consider that PAS granulation is a sine qua non, and this view is accepted by Niemi and Kormano (1964) as valid in the rat; Baillie (1961) added sudanophilia to his criteria of identification of murine Leydig cells. Baillie et al. (1965) have pointed out that intertubular cells in the human foetal testis exhibit histochemical evidence of steroid production long before they assume the morphological characteristics of mature Leydig tissue. In a sense, therefore, these observations serve as a precedent for the observed histochemical evidence of steroidogenesis in the apparently histologically typical fibroblasts associated with the mouse rete.

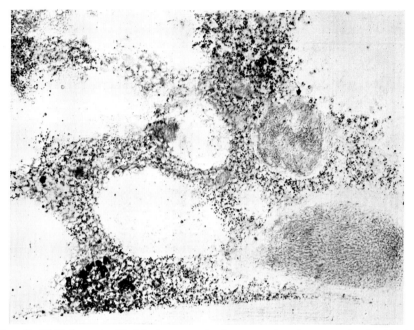

FIG. 42. 3β-Hydroxysteroid dehydrogenase in the connective tissue associated with the mouse rete testis. Sperm plugs can be seen in two tubuli recti. × 150.

IV. THE DUCTUS EPIDIDYMIS

The epididymis comprises an extensively convoluted tube or duct, and immature non-motile spermatozoa produced by the testis undergo the progressive anatomical, functional and biochemical changes which constitute maturation as they pass along the epididymis. Histochemically, the epididymis comprises of two active cell populations, namely spermatozoa, and the epithelial cells lining the duct of the epididymis. Both types exhibit considerable hydroxysteroid dehydrogenase activity, and are best considered separately. At the time of writing only the hamster epididymis has been fully investigated, and the following account is based entirely on the hamster results.

The spermatozoa in the epididymis are most numerous in the cauda epididymis, where they form masses of cells entirely filling the ducts of the epididymis. In the caput and body of the epididymis spermatozoa are more variable and are frequently difficult to find. The spermatozoa possess 3α-, 16α-, 16β- and 17β-hydroxysteroid dehydrogenases, and the activity of these enzymes (Fig. 43) increases steadily in activity as the spermatozoa pass distally along the epididymal duct. It would therefore appear that sperm maturation involves a progressive increase in ability to metabolize 3α-, 16α-, 16β- and 17β-hydroxysteroids, and this is in keeping with the growing bio-chemical evidence of steroid metabolism in spermatozoa (Schaffenburg and

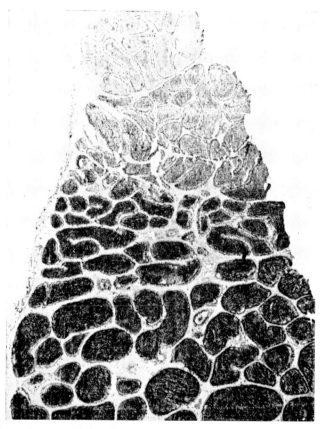

FIG. 43. 16β-Hydroxysteroid dehydrogenase activity in hamster spermatozoa in the cauda epididymidis. Note the great increase in activity as the sperm pass distally. A 16β-hydroxy-androgen was used as substrate, and it will be seen that the epididymal epithelium appears to be unable to dehydrogenate 16β-hydroxyandrogens. × 30.

McCullagh, 1954; Lofts and Marshall, 1959; Dirscherl and Breuer, 1963; Scott *et al.*, 1963; Hathaway and West, 1964; Mounib, 1964; Seamark and White, 1964; Christensen and Mason, 1965). Precisely how such a metabolic change fits maturing spermatozoa for their future environment is unclear. In assessing the increase in hydroxysteroid dehydrogenase activity in the epididymis as the spermatozoa pass distally, one must bear in mind the fact that the spermatozoa become compactly arranged and this could account for the changes seen in Fig. 43.

Two further points remain to be made in relation to hydroxysteroid dehydrogenase activity in the spermatozoa. First, the 3α-hydroxysteroid dehydrogenase present in spermatozoa is able to dehydrogenate both 5α- and 5β-steroids, unlike the enzyme in the epithelium (see below) of the cauda epididymidis which is specific for 3α-hydroxy-5β-steroids; similarly, the 16β-hydroxysteroid dehydrogenase in the spermatozoa can dehydrogenate both 16β-hydroxyandrogens and 16β-hydroxyoestrogens, and the enzyme found in the epididymal epithelium is specific for 16β-hydroxyoestrogens. This point will be considered further below. The second point of interest with respect to the activity noted in epididymal spermatozoa is the observation of Baillie and Mack (1966) that in adult human seminiferous tubules 3α-, 16β- and 17β-hydroxysteroids consistently give traces of formazan deposition. The epididymal results suggest that this enzymic activity in the testis may be located in the maturing spermatids rather than in the Sertoli cells.

With regard to the epithelium of the epididymal duct, it is now possible to infer extensive steroid metabolism throughout its length. A 16β-hydroxysteroid dehydrogenase, apparently specific for oestrogens, occurs in the epididymal epithelium from the testis to the vas deferens and appears to be a characteristic of hamster epididymal epithelium. Other hydroxysteroid dehydrogenases also occur in the epididymal epithelium but they are distributed in precise and well-defined zones. The epididymal zonation revealed by hydroxysteroid dehydrogenases is as follows.

The initial segment, whose epithelium has, as has all epididymal epithelium, strong 16β-hydroxysteroid dehydrogenase activity specific for steroids with an aromatic A-ring. No other hydroxysteroid dehydrogenases occur in this zone.

Zone 1 which comprises the initial few tubules of the caput epididymis and whose epithelium is unreactive, apart from the 16β-hydroxysteroid dehydrogenase common to all epididymal zones.

Zone 2 is characterized by weak epithelial 11β-hydroxysteroid dehydrogenase in addition to the usual 16β-hydroxysteroid dehydrogenase. The substrate of choice is cortisol.

Zone 3 is an area of intense cortisol utilization in the caput epididymis immediately distal to zone 2.

Zone 4 accounts for the remaining half or so of the caput epididymis together with the upper part of the body of the epididymis, and has only epithelial 16β-hydroxysteroid dehydrogenase demonstrable.

Zone 5 corresponds with the caudal part of the body of the epididymis and is characterized by the presence in the epithelium of an oestradiol-17β-hydroxysteroid dehydrogenase. Testosterone is not dehydrogenated by the epithelium in this zone.

Zone 6 represents the proximal quarter or so of the cauda epididymis and is unreactive, apart from the widespread 16β-hydroxysteroid dehydrogenase mentioned above.

Zone 7 (Fig. 45) is an area of small tubules in the cauda epididymis characterized by moderate cortisol utilization. It is immediately succeeded by

Zone 8 (Fig. 45), which is an area of intense epithelial utilization of cortisol.
Weak 3α-hydroxysteroid dehydrogenase is also present.

Zone 9 is the terminal zone of the epididymis (Fig. 45) and is occupied by
large sperm-filled ducts. The epithelium of these ducts exhibits 3α-, 11β-, 16α-
and 16β-hydroxysteroid dehydrogenases (Figs. 45, 46, 47). The 3α-hydroxy-
steroid dehydrogenase is specific for 5β-steroids; the 11β-hydroxysteroid
dehydrogenase is almost cortisol-specific; the 16α- and 16β-hydroxysteroid
dehydrogenases are apparently specific for steroids with an aromatic A-ring.
This pattern of epithelial activity continues into the vas deferens for a short
distance.

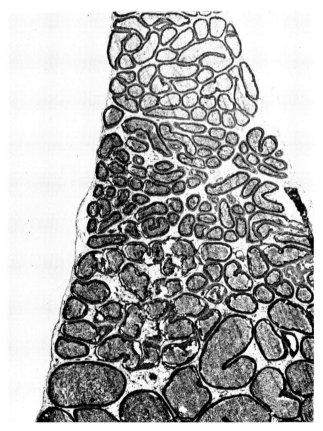

FIG. 44. A 16β-hydroxysteroid dehydrogenase specific for 16β-hydroxyoestrogens is present
in the epithelium of the hamster epididymis throughout its length. Notice also the increase
in activity of 16β-hydroxysteroid dehydrogenase in the spermatozoa as they pass distally.
Compare with Fig. 43. ×30.

The functional significance of this striking zonation is difficult to interpret. Steroids presumably influence maturation of the spermatozoa as they pass down the epididymis, but whether the hydroxysteroid dehydrogenases noted in different zones reflect steroid transport across the epithelium at different points or merely denote steroid control of the secretory activity of the epididymal epithelium remains to be determined. Electrolyte changes have been demonstrated in epididymal fluid as it traverses the duct, and it is tempting to implicate the two cortisol-using zones in the caput and cauda with the regulation of the sodium and potassium content of the epididymal fluid.

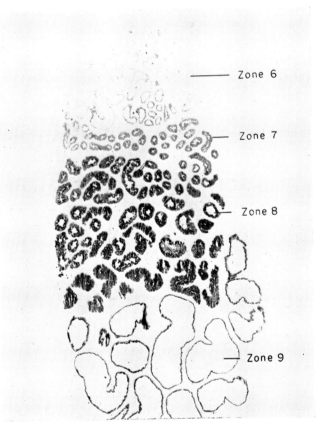

FIG. 45. Histochemical utilization of cortisol by zones 7, 8 and 9 of the epididymis. × 30.

Apart from the significance of the results obtained in the epididymis in considering the problem of specificity (p. 20), several biochemical conclusions can be drawn from the findings. First, in zones 8 and 9 it is clear that the epithelium possesses a 3α-hydroxysteroid dehydrogenase which is so stereo-

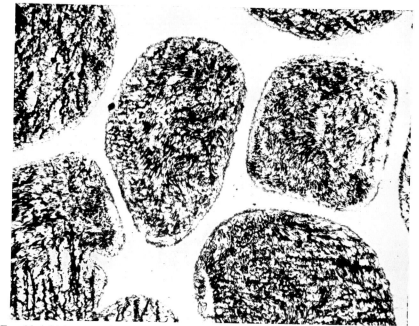

FIG. 46. A high-power view of zone 9 of the epididymis showing histochemical utilization of a 5α-3α-hydroxysteroid. Compare with Fig. 47. × 130.

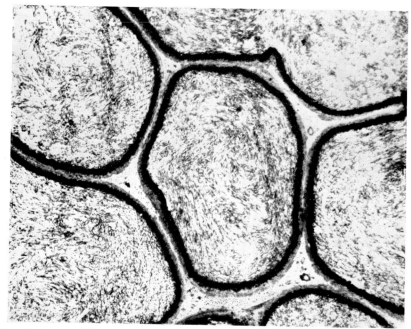

FIG. 47. Intense 5β-3α-hydroxysteroid dehydrogenase in the epithelium of zone 9 of the epididymis. Compare with Fig. 46. × 150.

specific as to merit the terminology 5β-3α-hydroxysteroid dehydrogenase. Moreover, comparison of Figs. 46 and 47 makes it quite clear that the epithelium and spermatozoa together of the distal part of the cauda epididymidis possess at least two different 3α-hydroxysteroid dehydrogenases. One is precisely defined by the term 5β-3α-hydroxysteroid dehydrogenase and

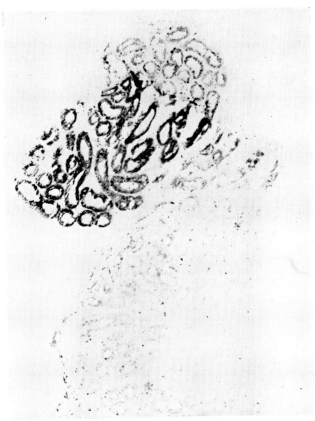

Fig. 48. Histochemical utilization of cortisol by zones 1 to 5 of the hamster epididymis. × 40.

is confined to the epithelium. The other in the spermatozoa, utilizes both 5α- and 5β-steroids, and may either be a less specific 3α-hydroxysteroid dehydrogenase capable of attacking 5α- and 5β-steroids or, possibly, may represent a mixture of two specific enzymes. In the same way the epididymal epithelium possesses a 16β-hydroxysteroid dehydrogenase which selectively utilizes steroids having an aromatic A-ring; the 16β-hydroxysteroid dehydrogenase demonstrable in the spermatozoa is either a mixture of enzymes or a less specific enzyme capable of dehydrogenating the 16β-hydroxyl group of both androgens and oestrogens.

REFERENCES

Aakvaag, A., Hagen, A. A. and Eik-Nes, K. B. (1964). Biosynthesis *in vivo* of testosterone and Δ^4-androstenedione from dehydroepiandrosterone-sodium sulfate by the canine testis and ovary. *Biochim. Biophys. Acta.* **86**, 622–627.

Acevedo, H. F., Axelrod, L. R., Ishikawa, E. and Takaki, F. (1963). Studies in fetal metabolism. II. Metabolism of progesterone-4-C^{14} and pregnenolone-7-H^3 in human fetal testes. *J. Clin. Endocrinol.* **23**, 885–890.

Arvy, L. (1962a). Action de l'hormone gonadotrope choriale sur quelques activités enzymatiques testiculaires chez le Rat. *Compt. Rend.* **255**, 1532–1534.

Arvy, L. (1962b). Présence d'une activite stéroïdo-3β-ol-deshydrogénasique chez quelques sauropsides. *Compt. Rend.* **255**, 1803–1804.

Baillie, A. H. (1961). Observations on the growth and histochemistry of the Leydig tissue in the postnatal prepubertal mouse testis. *J. Anat. (London)* **95**, 357–370.

Baillie A. H. (1965). 3β-Hydroxysteroid dehydrogenase activity in the foetal mouse testis. *J. Anat. (London)* **99**, 507–512.

Baillie, A. H. and Griffiths, K. (1964). 3β-Hydroxysteroid dehydrogenase activity in the mouse Leydig cell. *J. Endocrinol.* **29**, 9–17.

Baillie, A. H. and Griffiths, K. (1965a). 3β-Hydroxysteroid dehydrogenase in the foetal mouse Leydig cell. *J. Endocrinol.* **31**, 63–66.

Baillie, A. H. and Griffiths, K. (1965b). Further observations on 3β-hydroxysteroid dehydrogenase activity in the mouse Leydig cell. *J. Endocrinol.* **31**, 207–215.

Baillie, A. H. and Mack, W. S. (1966). Hydroxysteroid dehydrogenases in normal and abnormal human testes. *J. Endocrinol.* **35**, 239–248.

Baillie, A. H., Niemi, M. and Ikonen, M. (1965a). 3β-Hydroxysteroid dehydrogenase activity in the human foetal testis. *Acta Endocrinol.* **48**, 429–438.

Baillie, A. H., Calman, K. C., Ferguson, M. M. and Hart, D. McK. (1965b). Histochemical demonstration of 20β-hydroxysteroid dehydrogenase. *J. Endocrinol.* **32**, 337–339.

Baillie, A. H., Calman, K. C., Ferguson, M. M. and Hart, D. McK. (1966). Histochemical utilisation of 3α-, 6β-, 11α-, 12α-, 16α-, 16β-, 17α-, 21- and 24-hydroxysteroids. *J. Endocrinol.* **34**, 1–12.

Baillie, A. H., Ferguson, M. M., Calman, K. C. and Hart, D. McK. (1965c). Histochemical demonstration of 11β-hydroxysteroid dehydrogenase. *J. Endocrinol.* **33**, 119–125.

Berthrong, M., Goodwin, W. E. and Scott, W. W. (1949). Estrogen production by the testis. *J. Clin. Endocrinol.* **9**, 579–592.

Beyer, K. F. and Samuels, L. T. (1956). Distribution of steroid-3β-ol dehydrogenase in cellular structures of the adrenal gland. *J. Biol. Chem.* **219**, 69.

Botte, V. (1963). *Ist. Sci. Camerino* **4**, 205–209.

Breuer, H. and Nocke, L. (1959). Formation of estriol-3, 16β, 17α by liver tissue *in vitro*. *Biochim. Biophys. Acta* **36**, 271–272.

Breuer, H., Nocke, L. and Knuppen, R. (1958). 6β-Hydroxylierung von Oestrogenen in der Rattenleber. *Naturwissenschaften* **45**, 397.

Brinck-Johnsen, T. and Eik-Nes, K. (1957). Effect of human chorionic gonadotropin on the secretion of testosterone and 4-androstene-3, 17-dione by the canine testis. *Endocrinology* **61**, 676–683.

Cavallero, C., Martinazzi, M., Baroni, C. and Magrini, U. (1963). Pituitary control of mouse testis in hereditary dwarfism: histological and cytochemical observations. *Gen. Comp. Endocrinol.* **3**, 636–643.

Cavallero, C., Magrini, U., Deuepiane, M. and Cizelj, T. (1965). Etude histochimique du cortex surrénalien et du testicule chez le foetus humain. *Ann. d' Endocrinol. (Paris)* **26**, 409–418.

Certain, P., Collenot, G., Collenot, A., and Ozon, R. (1964). Mise en évidence biochimique et histochimique d'une Δ⁵-3β-hydroxysteroide déshydrogénase dans le testicule du Triton *Pleurodeles waltlii* Michah. *Compt. Rend. Soc. Biol.* **158**, 1040–1043.

Chieffi, G. (1964). Distribution of cholesterol and Δ⁵-3β-hydroxysteroid dehydrogenase in chick embryo gonad. *Ric. Sci. (Biol.)* **5**, 77–84.

Chieffi, G. and Botte, V. (1963). Osservazione istochimiche sull' attivita della steroide-3β-olo-deidrogenasi sull' interenale e nelle gonadi di girini e adulti di Rana esculenta. *Riv. Istoch. Norm. Pat.* **91**, 172–174.

Chieffi, G., Botte, V. and Visca, T. (1963). *Acta Med. Romana* **1**, 1–9.

Christensen, A. K. and Mason, N. R. (1965). Comparative ability of seminiferous tubules and interstitial tissue of rat testes to synthesis and androgens from progesterone-4-¹⁴C *in vitro*. *Endocrinology* **76**, 646–656.

Cole, H. H., Hart, G. H., Lyons, W. R. and Catchpole, H. R. (1933). The development and hormonal content of fetal horse gonads. *Anat. Record* **56**, 275–293

Collenot., A. and Ozon., R. (1964). Mises en évidence biochimique et histochimique d'une Δ⁵-3β-hydroxysteroide déshydrogenase dans le testicule de scylliarhinus canicula L. *Bull. Soc. Zool. France* **89**.

Deane, H. W. and Rubin, B. L. (1965). *Arch. Anat. Microscop. Morphol. Exptl.* (Quoted by Maeir, 1965).

Della Corte, F., Botte, V. and Chieffi, G. (1961). Ricerca istochimica dell' attivita della steroide-3β-olo-deidrogenasi nel testicolo di Terpedo marmerata Risso e di Scyliarhinus stelloris (L). *Atti. Soc. Peleritana Sci. Fis. Mat. Nat.* **7**, 393–397.

Della Corte, F., Galgano, M. and Cosenza, L. (1962). *Arch. Zool. Ital.* **47**, 353–363.

Dirscherl, W. and Breuer, H. (1963). Isolierung von dehydroepiandrosteron aus menschlichen sperma. *Acta Endocrinol.* **44**, 403–408.

Dorfman, R. I., Forchielli, E. and Gut, M. (1963). *Rec. Progr. Horm. Res.* **19**, 251.

Engel, L. L. and Langer, L. J. (1961). Biochemistry of steroid hormones. *Ann. Rev. Biochem.* **30**, 499–524.

Ewald, W., Werbin, H. and Chaikoff, I. L. (1964). Evidence of two substrate specific Δ⁵-3-ketosteroid isomerases in beef adrenal glands and their separation from 3β-hydroxysteroid dehydrogenase. *Biochem. Biophys. Acta.* **81**, 199–201.

Fuhrmann, K. (1963). Histochemische untersuchungen uber Hydroxysteroid Dehydrogenase-Aktivität in Nebennieren und Eierstöcken von Ratten und Kaninchen. *Arch. Gynaekol.* **197**, 583–600.

Gillman, J. (1948). The development of the gonads in man, with a consideration of the role of foetal endocrines and the histogenesis of ovarian tumours. *Carnegie Inst. Wash. Publ. Contrib. Embryol.* **210**, 81–131.

Goldberg, B., Jones, G. E. S. and Borkowf, H. I. (1964). A histochemical study of substrate specificity of the steroid 3β-ol dehydrogenase and isomerase systems in human ovary and testis. *J. Histochem. Cytochem.* **12**, 880–889.

Goldberg, B., Jones, G. E. S., Turner, D. A., Sarlos, I. J. and Horton, H. E. H. (1963). Steroid 3β-ol-dehydrogenase activity in human endocrine tissues. *Am. J. Obstet. Gynecol.* **86**, 349–359.

Goldman, A. S., Yakovac, W. C. and Bongiovanni, A. M. (1965). Persistent effects of a synthetic androstene derivative on activities of 3β-Hydroxysteroid dehydrogenase and glucose-6-phosphate dehydrogenase in rats. *Endocrinology* **77**, 1105–1118.

Goldman, A. S., Yakovac, W. C. and Bongiovanni, A. M. (1966). Development of activity of 3β-hydroxysteroid dehydrogenase in human fetal tissues and in two anencephalic newborns. *J. Clin. Endocrinol.* **26**, 14–22.

Goldstein, M., Gut, M. and Dorfman, R. (1960). Conversion of pregnenolone to dehydroepiandrosterone. *Biochem. Biophys. Acta* **38**, 190.

Gower, D. B. and Haslewood, G. A. D. (1961). Biosynthesis of androst-16-en-3α-ol from acetate by testicular slices. *J. Endocrinol.* **23**, 253–260.

Griffiths, K. and Grant, J. K. (1962). Steroid biosynthesis in a case of testicular feminization. *Biochem. J.* **84**, 22p.

Hagen, A. A. and Eik-Nes, K. B. (1964). Conversion of 17β-hydroxypregnenolone to 17β-hydroxyprogesterone by the canine testis *in vivo*. *Biochim. Biophys. Acta.* **86**, 372–379.

Hart, D. McK., Baillie, A. H., Calman, K. C. and Ferguson, M. M. (1966a). Hydroxysteroid dehydrogenose development in mouse adrenad and gonads. *J. Anat. (London)* (in press).

Hart, D. McK., Calman, K. C., Ferguson, M. M., Niemi, M. and Baillie, A. H. (1966b). Hydroxysteroid dehydrogenase activity in human foetal gonads. M.D. Thesis. Hart. Glasgow University.

Hathaway, R. R. and West, C. D. (1964). Conversion of 17β-Estradiol to estrone by spermatozoa of dogs and men. *Endocrinology* **75**, 616–618.

Hitzeman, J. W. (1962). Development of enzymic activity in the Leydig cells of the mouse testis. *Anat. Record.* **143**, 351–361.

Hofmann, F. G. (1962). The concerted action upon a common substrate of steroid hydroxylases from the adrenal cortex and the testis. *Biochem. Biophys. Acta.* **58**, 343–348.

Hooker, C. W. (1948). The biology of the interstitial cells of the testis. *Recent Progr. Hormone Res.* **3**, 173–196.

Hubener, H. J. and Sahrholtz, F. G. (1960). 20β-Hydroxysteroid dehydrogenase. *Biochem. Z.* **333**, 95–105.

Hubener, H. J., Sahrholtz, F. G., Schmidt-Thome, J., Nesemann, G. and Junk, R. (1959). 20β-Hydroxysteroid dehydrogenase, ein neues kristallines Enzym. *Biochim. Biophys. Acta.* **35**, 270–272.

Huggins, C. and Moulder, P. V. (1945). Estrogen production by Sertoli cell tumors of the testis. *Cancer Res.* **5**, 510–514.

Jirasek, J. E. and Raboch, J. (1963). Histochemical study of testicular material from patients with various disorders. *Fertility Sterility* **14**, 237–245.

Koch, F. C. (1944). The steroids. *Ann. Rev. Biochem.* **13**, 263–294.

Kruskemper, H. L., Forchielli, E. and Ringold, H. J. (1964). Δ⁵-3-keto isomerase; specificity and inhibition studies in bovine adrenal homogenate fractions and distribution in rat tissues. *Steroids* **3**, 295–309.

Leeson, T. S. (1962). Electron microscopy of the rete testis of the rat. *Anat. Record.* **144**, 57–61.

Levitz, M., Spitzer, T. R. and Twombly, G. G. (1958). Interconversions of 16-

oxygenated oestrogens. I. The synthesis of estriol-16-C^{14} and its metabolism in man. *J. Biol. Chem.* **231**, 787–797.

Lipsett, M. B. and Hökfelt, B. (1961). Conversion of 17α-hydroxypregnenolone to cortisol. *Experientia* **17**, 449.

Lofts, B. and Marshall, A. J. (1959). The post-nuptial occurrence of progestins in the seminiferous tubules of birds. *J. Endocrinol.* **19**, 16–21.

Lupo, C. and Chieffi, G. (1963). Ormoni sersuali e attivita steroide-3β-olodeidrogenasua del testicolo di *Morane lubrax*. *Atti Acad. Nuzl. Lincei Rend., Classe Sci. Fis., Mat. Nat.* **24**, 443–446.

Maeir, D. (1965). Species variation in testicular hydroxysteroid dehydrogenase activity; absence of activity in primate Leydig cells. *Endocrinology* **76**, 463–469.

Magrini, U. (1965). Histoenzymatic observations on the human fetal testicle. *Minerva. Pediat.* **17**, 556–558.

Magrini, U. and Martinazzi, M. (1964). Enzyme histochemistry of steroidogenesis in Leydig cell of pituitary dwarf mice. In: *Research on Steroids*, **1**, 295–298.

Mancini, R. E., Vilar, O., Lavieri, J. E., Andrada, J. A. and Heinrich, J. J. (1963). Development of Leydig cells in the normal human testis. *Am. J. Anat.* **112**, 203–214.

Mosebach, K. O., Dirscherl, W. and El-Attar, T. (1963). Die initiale Metaboliserung von Testosteran-4-14C in der ratte. *Acta Endochrinol* **44**, 416–429.

Mounib, M. S. (1964). Effects of certain hormones on the metabolism of bull spermatozoa. *Acta Endocrinol.* **45**, 631–640.

Mulrow, P. H., Cohn, G. L. and Kuljian, A. (1962). Conversion of 17-hydroxypregnenolone to cortisol. *Experientia* **17**, 449.

Narbaitz, R. and Kolodny, L. (1964). Δ^5, 3β-OH-steroid dehydrogenase in differentiating *chick* gonads. *Z. Zellforsch.* **63**, 612–617.

Neher, R. and Wettstein, A. (1960). Occurrence of Δ^5-3β-hydroxysteroids in adrenal and testicular tissue. *Acta Endocrinol* **35**, 1–7.

Niemi, M. and Ikonen, M. (1962). Histochemistry of the Leydig cells in the postnatal prepubertal testis of the rat. *Endocrinology* **72**, 443–448.

Niemi, M. and Kormano, M. (1964). Cyclical changes in and significance of lipids and acid phosphatase activity in the seminiferous tubules of the rat testis. *Anat. Record.* **151**, 159–170.

Pearson, B. and Grose, F. (1959a). Histochemical study of some DPNH and DPN dependent dehydrogenases. *Federation Proc.* **18**, 499.

Pearson, B. and Grose, F. (1959b). Histochemical demonstration of 17β-hydroxysteroid dehydrogenase by use of a tetrazolium salt. *Proc. Soc. Exptl. Biol. Med.* **100**, 636–638.

Prelog, V. and Ruzicka, L. (1944). Untersuchungen uber organextrakte (v) Mitteilung. Uber zwei moschufartig reichende steroide aus schweinetestes-extrakten. *Helv. Chim. Acta.* **27**, 61–66.

Price, D., Ortiz, E. and Deane, H. W. (1964). The presence of Δ^5-3β-hydroxysteroid dehydrogenase in fetal guinea pig testes and adrenal glands. *Amer. Zool.* **4**, No. 4.

Roosen-Runge, E. C. and Anderson, D. (1959). The development of the interstitial cells in the testis of the albino rat. *Acta Anat.* **37**, 125–137.

Rosner, J. G., Horita, S. and Forsham, P. (1964). Androstenediol, a probable intermediate in the *in vitro* conversion of Dehydroepiandrosterone to testosterone by the rabbit testis. *Endocrinology* **75**, 299–303.

Samuels, L. T. and Helmreich, M. L. (1956). The influence of chorionic gonadotropin on the 3β-ol dehydrogenase activity of testes and adrenals. *Endocrinology* **58**, 435–442.

Samuels, L., Helmreich, M. L., Lasater, M. and Reich, M. (1951). An enzyme in endocrine tissues which oxidises Δ^5-3β-hydroxysteroids to α, β unsaturated ketones. *Science* **113**, 490.

Savard, K. and Dorfman, R. I. (1954). *Rev. Can. Biol.* **13**, 495 (Abstract).

Savard, K. and Goldzieher, J. W. (1960). Biosynthesis of steroids in stallion testis tissue. *Endocrinology* **66**, 617–624.

Savard, K., Dorfman, R. I., Baggett, B., Fielding, L. L., Engel, L. L., McPherson, H. T., Lister, L. M., Johnson, D. S., Hamblen, E. C. and Engel, F. L. (1960). Clinical morphological and biochemical studies of a virilizing tumour in the testis. *J. Clin. Invest.* **39**, 534–553.

Schaffenburg, C. A. and McCullagh, E. P. (1954). Studies in sperm hormones: demonstration of oestrogenic activity. *Endocrinology* **54**, 296–302.

Scott, T. W., Baggett, B. and White, I. G. (1963). Metabolism of testosterone by semen and effect of testosterone on oxidative metabolism of spermatozoa. *Aust. J. Exptl. Biol. Med. Sci.* **41**, 363.

Seamark, R. F. and White, I. G. (1964). The metabolism of steroid hormones in semen. *J. Endrocrinol.* **30**, 307–321.

Shikita, M. and Tamaoki, B. (1965). 20α-Hydroxysteroid dehydrogenase of testes. *Biochemistry* **4**, 1189–1195.

Smith, E. R., Breuer, H. and Genrieffers, H. (1964). A study of the steroid metabolism of an interstitial cell tumour of the testis. *Biochem. J.* **93**, 583–587.

Stanley, H., Chieffi, G. and Botte, V. (1965). Histological and histochemical observations on the testis of *Gobius pagellanus*. *Z. Zellforsch.* **65**, 350–362.

Talalay, P. (1965). Enzymic mechanisms in steroid biochemistry. *Ann. Rev. Biochem.* **34**, 347–380

Treves, N. (1958). Gynecomastia; the origins of mammary swelling in the male: an analysis of 406 patients with breast hypertrophy, 525 with testicular tumors and 13 with adrenal neoplasms. *Cancer* **11**, 1083.

Ulstrom, R. A., Colle, E., Burley, J. and Gunville, R. (1960). Adrenocortical steroid metabolism in newborn infants. II. Urinary excretion of 6β-hydroxy cortisol and other polar metabolites. *J. Clin. Endocrinol.* **20**, 1080.

Wattenberg, L. W. (1958). Microscopic histochemical demonstration of steroid-3β-ol dehydrogenase in tissue sections. *J. Histochem. Cytochem.* **6**, 225–232.

Weliky, I. and Engel, L. L. (1962). Conversion *in vitro* of 17-hydroxypregnenolone to cortisol by a human adrenal tumor. *J. Biol. Chem.* **237**, 2089.

Weliky, I. and Engel, L. L. (1963). Metabolism of progesterone-4-C^{14} and pregnenolone-7-H^3 by human adrenal tissue. *J. Biol. Chem.* **238**, 1302.

Yaron, Z. (1966). Demonstration of 3β-hydroxysteroid dehydrogenase in the testis of *Tilapia mossambica*. *J. Endocrinol.* **34**, 127–128.

Zander, J., Forbes, T. R., Von Munstermann, A. M. and Neher, R. (1960). Δ^4-3-ketopregnene-20α-ol and Δ^4-3-ketopregnene-20β-ol, two naturally occurring metabolites of progesterone, isolation, identification; biologic activity and concentration in human tissues. *J. Clin. Endocrinol.* **18**, 337–353.

CHAPTER 5

The Ovary

I. ENZYMES

Numerous histochemical tests have been applied to the ovary in the hope of localizing various types of lipids and possibly steroids. Although subjecting a tissue to this range of reactions may provide some indication of steroid metabolism, it is clear that many of these techniques are not highly specific. Nevertheless it was concluded from these earlier investigations on the ovary (Dempsey and Basset, 1943; McKay and Robinson, 1947; Claesson and Hillarp, 1947a, b; Everett, 1947; Deane, 1952; Claesson, 1954) that the principal sites of steroid metabolism were the theca interna, interstitial tissue, corpora lutea and granulosa of atretic follicles. The histochemical distribution of the hydroxysteroid dehydrogenases in the ovary is in many ways in keeping with the inferences drawn from earlier lipid studies, but the precise nature of the technique has clarified some aspects of ovarian steroid metabolism.

The histochemical demonstration of hydroxysteroid dehydrogenases depends on the presence of a diaphorase to transfer hydrogen from the reduced pyridine nucleotide to a tetrazolium salt. Although both NAD and NADP diaphorase are virtually ubiquitous in the ovary, they do exhibit quantitative differences in activity. NAD diaphorase is intensely active in the theca interna, interstitial tissue, corpora lutea, granulosa of atretic follicles, blood vessel walls and germinal epithelium; a much weaker reaction is seen in normal healthy granulosa and connective tissue stroma. The distribution of

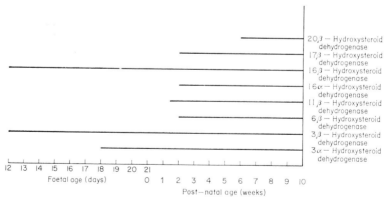

FIG. 49. Histogram showing times of appearance of hydroxysteroid dehydrogenase in developing mouse ovaries.

72

NADP diaphorase is essentially the same but with one striking difference in the rat at least; the germinal epithelium, which is rich in NAD diaphorase (M. M. Ferguson, unpublished), almost entirely lacks NADP diaphorase.

TABLE 5

Distribution of 3α-hydroxysteroid dehydrogenase in the ovary

Species	Substrate	Distribution	Investigators
Rat	Pregnanediol	Not demonstrated	Pearson and Grose (1959a)
Human	Androstanediol	Not demonstrated	Goldberg et al. (1964)
	Androsterone		
	Aetiocholanolone		
Rat	Androsterone	T.I., I.T., C.L.	Goldman et al. (1965)
Mouse	Androsterone	a.O., a.G., T.I., I.T., C.L.	Baillie et al. (1966)
	Aetiocholanolone	a.O., a.G., T.I., I.T., C.L.	
Mouse (foetal and Postnatal)	Androsterone	a.O., a.G., T.I., I.T., C.L.	Hart et al. (1966)
	Aetiocholanolone	a.O., a.G., T.I., I.T., C.L.	
Rat	Androsterone[a]	a.O., a.G., T.I., I.T., C.L.	M. M. Ferguson (unpublished)
Mouse	Aetiocholanolone	a.G., T.I., I.T., C.L.	
	Androsterone	a.G., T.I., I.T., C.L.	
Hamster	Aetiocholanolone	a.G., T.I., I.T., C.L.	
	Androsterone	a.G., T.I., I.T., C.L.	
	Aetiocholanolone	a.G., T.I., I.T., C.L.	
Guinea-pig	Androsterone	C.L.	
	Aetiocholanolone	C.L.	
Rabbit	Androsterone	I.T.	
	Aetiocholanolone	I.T.	
Fowl	Androsterone	G., T.I.	
	Aetiocholanolone	G., T.I.	
Human	Androsterone	T.I., C.L.	M. M. Ferguson and D. McK. Hart (unpublished)
	Aetiocholanolone	T.I., C.L.	

[a] A particularly intense reaction occurred in rat corpora lutea using androsterone as substrate.

a.O. = Atretic ova. G. = Normal granulosa. a.G. = Atretic granulosa. T.I. = Theca interna. I.T. = Interstitial tissue. C.L. = Corpora lutea.

A. 3α-HYDROXYSTEROID DEHYDROGENASE

One or two earlier workers (Table 5) failed to demonstrate 3α-hydroxy-steroid dehydrogenase activity in rodent and human ovary, perhaps for technical reasons; but we have found the enzyme consistently in most ovarian tissues, normal granulosa and germinal epithelium excepted. The enzyme is first histochemically present in the mouse ovary (Fig. 49) during foetal life (Hart *et al.*, 1966a), but is absent from foetal human ovaries at the twentieth week of gestation (Hart *et al.*, 1966b). In the foetal rodent, ovarian 3α-hydroxysteroid dehydrogenase is invariably much weaker than testicular 3α-hydroxysteroid dehydrogenase at a comparable stage of development, and this may reflect the fact that, whereas androgens are required to secure male differentiation, steroids of placental or maternal origin suffice to induce female differentiation (Price and Pannabecker, 1956; Diczfalusy *et al.*, 1961).

In biochemical systems both the 5α- and 5β-isomers serve as substrates for 3α-hydroxysteroid dehydrogenase (Tomkins, 1956); this is true of the weak 3α-hydroxysteroid dehydrogenase found histochemically in the theca interna

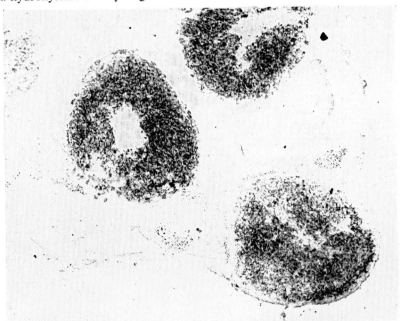

Fig. 50. Heavy deposit of diformazan in corpora lutea of rat ovary incubated with 3α-hydroxy-5α-androstan-17-one. × 70.

and interstitial tissue of the ovary. In the corpora lutea of the rat ovary, by contrast, there is a strong 3α-hydroxysteroid dehydrogenase which (Fig. 50) is stereo-specific, apparently, for the 5α-isomer (M. M. Ferguson, unpublished). The significance of this observation will be returned to in relation to steroid biosynthesis in the corpus luteum (p. 94).

TABLE 6(a)

Distribution of Δ^5-3β-hydroxysteroid dehydrogenase in the ovary

Species	Substrate	Distribution	Investigators
Rabbit	Pregnenolone and DHA	I.T.	Wattenberg (1958)
Human		C.L.	
Rat		I.T., C.L.	
Rat	DHA	a.G., T.I., I.T., C.L.	Levy et al. (1959a)
Mouse		a.G., T.I., I.T., C.L.	
Guinea-pig		a.G., T.I., I.T., C.L.	
Hamster		a.G., T.I., I.T., C.L.	
Rat	DHA	a.G., T.I., I.T., C.L.	Levy et al. (1959b)
Rat	DHA	a.G., T.I., I.T., C.L.	Deane et al. (1961)
Human	Pregnenolone and DHA	a.G., T.I., I.T., C.L.	Fuhrmann (1961)
Rat			
Dog			
Human	Pregnenolone and DHA	a.G., T.I., I.T., C.L.	Ikonen et al. (1961)
Rat	DHA	a.G., T.I., I.T., C.L.	Taylor (1961)
Human	Not known	Stein-Leventhal Ovaries	Acosta (1962), quoted by Goldberg et al. (1963)
			Botte and Del Bianco (1962)
Rat	DHA		Deane et al. (1962)
Human	DHA	a.G., T.I. C.L.	Botte (1963a)
Raja sp.	DHA		Botte (1963b)
Rana esculenta	DHA		Chieffi and Botte (1963)
Rat	Pregnenolone and DHA		Fuhrmann (1963)
Rabbit			
Human		Arrhenoblastoma and luteinized granulosa cell tumour. Not demonstrated in thecoma	Goldberg et al. (1963)
Human	DHA		Goldberg et al. (1963)

TABLE 6(*a*). Continued

Species	Substrate	Distribution	Investigators
Mouse	DHA	a.G., T.I., I.T., C.L.	Rubin *et al.* (1963)
Rat		a.G., T.I., I.T., C.L.	
Guinea-pig		a.G., T.I., I.T., C.L.	
Rabbit		T.I., I.T.	
Dog		Not demonstrated	
Cat		C.L.	
Sheep		C.L.	
Cow		C.L.	
Horse		C.L.	
Armadillo		Not demonstrated	
Rat (developing)	DHA	a.G., T.I., I.T., C.L.	Rubin *et al.* (1963a)
Rat			Turolla and Magrini (1963)
Human	Pregnenolone	T.I.	Goldberg *et al.* (1964)
	DHA	T.I.	
	3β, 17β-Dihydroxyandrost-4-ene	T.I.	
	3β, 17β-Dihydroxyandrost-5-ene	T.I.	
	3β, 17α-Dihydroxyandrost-4-ene	T.I.	
	3β, 20β-Dihydroxypregn-4-ene	T.I.	
	3β, 17α-Dihydroxypregn-5-ene-20-one	Not demonstrated	
Human	DHA	C.L.	Kern-Bontke (1964)
Chicken (developing)	DHA	Between medullary lacunae	Narbaitz and Kolodny (1964)
Guinea-pig (foetal)	DHA	Not demonstrated	Price *et al.* (1964)
Fowl	Pregnenolone	G., T.I.	Wyburn and Baillie (1964)
	17α-Hydroxypregnenolone	G., T.I.	
	DHA	G., T.I.	
	Androstenediol	G., T.I.	
Fish (mackerel)	DHA	Theca cells	Bara (1965)
Fowl	DHA	G., T.I.	Chieffi and Botte (1965)
		(Pre- and post-ovulatory follicles and atretic follicles)	

Species	Substrate	Activity	Reference
Mouse	Pregnenolone	a.G., T.I., I.T., C.L.	Ferguson (1965)
	17α-Hydroxypregnenolone	a.G., T.I., I.T., C.L.	
	DHA	a.G., T.I., I.T., C.L.	
	Androstenediol	a.G., T.I., I.T., C.L.	
Human	DHA	T.I., C.L.	Fienberg and Cohen*(1965)
Rat	DHA	T.I., I.T., C.L.	Goldman et al. (1965)
	Pregnenolone	T.I., I.T., C.L.	
	17α-Hydroxypregnenolone	T.I., I.T., C.L.	
Rat (developing)	DHA	T.I., I.T.	Presl et al. (1965)
Rat	DHA	a.G., T.I., I.T., C.L.	Rubin and Deane (1965)
Rat	DHA	a.G., T.I., I.T., C.L.	Rubin et al. (1965)
Rat	Cholesterol	Not demonstrated	M. M. Ferguson (unpublished)
Mouse	Pregnenolone	a.G., T.I., I.T., C.L.	
	17α-Hydroxypregnenolone	a.G., T.I., I.T., C.L.	
	DHA	a.G., T.I., I.T., C.L.	
Hamster	Pregnenolone	a.G., T.I., I.T., C.L.	
	DHA	a.G., T.I., I.T., C.L.	
Guinea-pig	Pregnenolone	a.G., T.I., I.T., C.L.	
	DHA	a.G., T.I., I.T., C.L.	
Rabbit	Pregnenolone	I.T.	
	DHA	I.T.	
Cow	Pregnenolone	C.L.	
	DHA	C.L.	
Sheep	Pregnenolone	C.L.	
	DHA	C.L.	
Pig	Pregnenolone	T.I.	
	DHA	T.I.	
Fowl	Pregnenolone	G., T.I.	
	DHA	G., T.I.	

TABLE 6(a). Continued

Species	Substrate	Distribution		Investigators
Frog	Pregnenolone	I.T.		
	DHA	I.T.		
Human	Cholesterol	Not demonstrated		M. M. Ferguson and D. McK. Hart (unpublished)
	Pregnenolone	T.I.	C.L.	
	17α-Hydroxypregnenolone	T.I.	C.L.	
	DHA	T.I.	C.L.	
Human (foetal)	DHA	Follicular cells		Goldman et al. (1966)
Mouse (developing)	DHA	a.G., T.I., I.T., C.L.		Hart et al. (1966)
Human (foetal)	DHA	Not demonstrated		Hart et al. (1966)

a.O. = Atretic ova. G. = Normal granulosa. a.G. = Atretic granulosa. T.I. = Theca interna. I.T. = Interstitial tissue. C.L. = Corpora lutea.

TABLE 6(b)

Distribution of 3β-hydroxysteroid dehydrogenase in the ovary

Species	Substrate	Distribution		Investigators
Human	Epiandrosterone	T.I.	C.L.	Goldberg et al. (1964)
	3β, 17β-Dihydroxyandrostane	T.I.	C.L.	
	3β, 20β-Dihydroxy-5α-pregnane		C.L.	M. M. Ferguson
Rat	3β-Hydroxy-5β-androstan-17-one	a.G., T.I., I.T., C.L.		(unpublished)
Mouse	3β-Hydroxy-5β-androstan-17-one	a.G., T.I., I.T., C.L.		
Hamster	3β-Hydroxy-5β-androstan-17-one	a.G., T.I., I.T., C.L.		
Guinea-pig	3β-Hydroxy-5β-androstan-17-one	a.G., T.I., I.T., C.L.		
Rabbit	3β-Hydroxy-5β-androstan-17-one	a.G., T.I., I.T.		
Sheep	3β-Hydroxy-5β-androstan-17-one	T.I.	C.L.	
Cow	3β-Hydroxy-5β-androstan-17-one	T.I.	C.L.	
Pig	3β-Hydroxy-5β-androstan-17-one	T.I.	C.L.	
Fowl	3β-Hydroxy-5β-androstan-17-one	G., T.I.		
Frog	3β-Hydroxy-5β-androstan-17-one	I.T.		
Human	3β-Hydroxy-5β-androstan-17-one	a.G., T.I.	C.L.	

G. = Normal granulosa. a.G. = Atretic granulosa. T.I. = Theca interna.
I.T. = Interstitial tissue. C.L. = Corpora lutea.

3α-Hydroxysteroid dehydrogenase has been ascribed a transhydrogenase function (Talalay, 1957; Baron *et al.*, 1963), and this may influence steroid biosynthesis either because of the role played by reduced NADP in steroid hydroxylations and reductions, or on account of the relationship of NAD–NADP hydrogen transfer to general energy production (Fig. 8).

B. Δ^5-3β-HYDROXYSTEROID DEHYDROGENASE

The ovarian distribution of Δ^5-3β-hydroxysteroid dehydrogenase, as recorded by various workers, is summarized in Table 6 (a). It will be seen that considerable species and individual variations occur. Although virtually all workers in this field of ovarian histochemistry have utilized only NAD as co-factor, Ferguson (unpublished observations) has noted that NAD and NADP serve equally well as co-factors in the rat ovary.

The indifferent gonad becomes recognizable as ovary in the female mouse on the twelfth day of foetal life, and weak Δ^5-3β-hydroxysteroid dehydrogenase is present at this stage (Figs. 49 and 51) (Hart *et al.*, 1966a). Other workers (Presl *et al.*, 1965) failed to find 3β-hydroxysteroid dehydrogenase in rat ovaries before the eighth day of post-natal life, and Hart *et al.* (1966b) could find no significant enzyme activity in human foetal ovaries up to the twentieth week of gestation. Although Goldman *et al.* (1966) found Δ^5-3β-

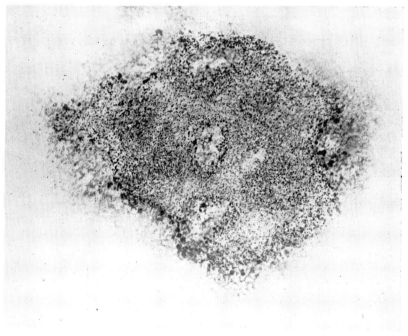

Fig. 51. Δ^5-3β-Hydroxysteroid dehydrogenase in mouse foetal ovary (18 days). $\times$ 200.

hydroxysteroid dehydrogenase in the ovaries of a 12 cm human foetus, we are unwilling to place any reliance on this observation on account of the 12–96 hr delay in freezing tissues after death (see p. 3).

Biochemical evidence exists for the biosynthesis and metabolism of steroids by the foetal ovary (Roberts and Warren, 1964; Bloch *et al.*, 1965), and the histochemical failure to demonstrate 3β-hydroxysteroid dehydrogenase in human foetal ovaries may reflect the threshold of activity of the histochemical techniques.

Extensive biochemical investigations have shown that the ovary has the capacity to convert acetate and cholesterol to pregnenolone, progesterone, 17α-hydroxypregnenolone, 17α-hydroxyprogesterone, DHA, androstenedione, androstenediol and testosterone (Wiest *et al.*, 1959; Ryan and Smith, 1961a, b, c, d; Savard *et al.*, 1961; Tamaoki and Pincus, 1961; Noall *et al.*, 1962; Depaoli and Eik-Nes, 1963; Forleo and Collins, 1964; Gospodarowicz, 1964; Ryan and Smith, 1965), the significance of which is illustrated in Fig. 10.

Histochemical results in rat ovary (M. M. Ferguson, unpublished) show that androstenediol and DHA are slightly better utilized than pregnenolone, but 17α-hydroxypregnenolone is a much less suitable substrate.

Goldberg *et al.* (1964) record formazan deposits in the human ovary incubated with DHA acetate, and Ferguson (1965) noted that a strong colour reaction could be demonstrated with pregnenolone acetate, DHA acetate and androstenediol diacetate in the various constituents of the rodent ovary. The activity distribution obtained with acetoxysteroids is identical with that observed with the free steroids. These findings could be explained by a steroid esterase in association with the dehydrogenase.

The sulphoxy derivatives of pregnenolone, and 17α-hydroxypregnenolone, exhibit a very poor reaction in the mouse ovary, and this is in marked contrast to the reactions observed with steroid sulphates in the testis.

C. 6β-HYDROXYSTEROID DEHYDROGENASE

The tissue distribution of ovarian 6β-hydroxysteroid dehydrogenase is

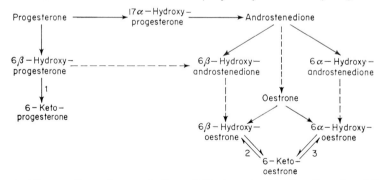

FIG. 52. Diagram illustrating metabolism of 6-hydroxysteroids. Reactions 1 and 2 are catalysed by 6β-hydroxysteroid dehydrogenase and reaction 3 by 6α-hydroxysteroid dehydrogenase.

TABLE 7

Demonstration of 6β-hydroxysteroid dehydrogenase in the ovary

Species	Substrate	Distribution	Investigators
Mouse	6β-Hydroxyprogesterone	a.O., a.G., T.I., I.T., C.L.	Baillie *et al.* (1966)
Rat	6β-Hydroxyprogesterone	a.G., T.I., I.T., C.L.	M. M. Ferguson (unpublished)
Mouse (developing)	6β-Hydroxyprogesterone	a.G., T.I., I.T., C.L.	Hart *et al.* (1966)

a.O. = Atretic ova. a.G. = Atretic granulosa. T.I. = Theca interna. I.T. = Interstitial tissue. C.L. = Corpora lutea.

TABLE 8

Demonstration of 11β-hydroxysteroid dehydrogenase in the ovary

Species	Substrate	Distribution	Investigators
Mouse	11β-Hydroxyprogesterone	a.G., T.I., I.T., C.L.	Baillie *et al.* (1965)
	11β-Hydroxyandrostenedione	a.G., T.I., I.T., C.L.	
	11β-Hydroxyoestrone	Not demonstrated	

a.G. = Atretic granulosa. T.I. = Theca interna. I.T. = Interstitial tissue. C.L. = Corpora lutea.

summarized in Table 7. Activity is weak and NAD-linked, and appears (Fig. 49) late in development (Hart *et al.*, 1966a). 6β-Hydroxyoestradiol has been isolated from equine follicular fluid (Short, 1962a, b; 1964), and on the basis of biochemical studies in other tissues it would seem that 6β-hydroxysteroid dehydrogenase is concerned in the metabolism of progesterone and oestrogens in the manner shown in Fig. 52; its precise role in the ovary, however, remains uncertain.

D. 11β-HYDROXYSTEROID DEHYDROGENASE

The distribution of 11β-hydroxysteroid dehydrogenase in the ovary is shown in Table 8.

M. M. Ferguson (unpublished) was unable to obtain a histochemical reaction with 11β-hydroxyandrostenedione in rat ovary, but it is known that rodent tissues are not capable of dehydrogenating 11β-hydroxysteroids as readily as human tissues (Koerner and Hellman, 1964), and this may explain the poor results.

11β-Hydroxysteroid dehydrogenase is responsible for the cortisol–cortisone reaction, and although cortisol has been isolated from the liquor folliculi of the mare (Short, 1962a, b) the significance of its occurrence in the ovary is obscure. An alternative role for the 11β-hydroxysteroid dehydrogenase in the ovary may be in the metabolism of 11β-hydroxyoestrogens and 11β-hydroxy-androgens. 11β-Hydroxyandrostenedione has been isolated from an ovarian interstitial cell tumour (Cohn and Mulrow, 1961), and in other tissues 11β-hydroxyoestrone has been synthesized from oestrone and cortisone (Chang and Dao, 1962; Knuppen and Breuer, 1962).

E. 16α-HYDROXYSTEROID DEHYDROGENASE

The tissue distribution of 16α-hydroxysteroid dehydrogenase in the ovary is shown in Table 9 and the murine age distribution in Fig. 49.

Both 16α-hydroxyprogesterone (Warren and Salhanick, 1961; Varangot and Cedard, 1962) and oestriol (Wotiz *et al.*, 1956; Layne and Marrian, 1958; Smith, 1960; Chieffi, 1962) have been isolated from ovarian tissue, and the principal role of 16α-hydroxysteroid dehydrogenase appears to be in oestrogen metabolism; it is illustrated in Fig. 53.

F. 16β-HYDROXYSTEROID DEHYDROGENASE

The distribution of 16β-hydroxysteroid dehydrogenase in the ovary is shown in Table 10.

An intense NAD-dependent 16β-hydroxysteroid dehydrogenase reaction occurs in the adult mouse ovary and can be found in the 12-day foetal mouse ovary. Ferguson (unpublished) also noted that NADP was a suitable co-factor in the rat and that the 3β, 16β-dihydroxyandrost-5-ene-3-methyl ether was better utilized that 16β-hydroxyoestrone.

TABLE 9

Demonstration of 16α-Hydroxysteroid dehydrogenase in the ovary

Species	Substrate	Distribution	Investigators
Mouse	16α-Hydroxyoestrone	a.O. T.I., I.T., C.L.	Baillie et al. (1966)
	16α-Hydroxyprogesterone	a.O. T.I., I.T., C.L.	
Rat	16α-Hydroxyoestrone	a.G., T.I., I.T., C.L.	M. M. Ferguson (unpublished)
Mouse	16α-Hydroxyoestrone	a.G., T.I., I.T., C.L.	
Hamster	16α-Hydroxyoestrone	I.T.	
Guinea-pig	16α-Hydroxyoestrone	C.L.	
Rabbit	16α-Hydroxyoestrone	I.T.	
Pig	16α-Hydroxyoestrone	C.L.	
Fowl	16α-Hydroxyoestrone	G., T.I.	
Human	16α-Hydroxyoestrone	C.L.	M. M. Ferguson and D. McK. Hart (unpublished)
Mouse (developing)	16α-Hydroxyprogesterone	a.G., T.I., I.T., C.L., G.E.	Hart et al. (1966)

a.O. = Atretic ova. G. = Normal granulosa. a.G. = Atretic granulosa. T.I. = Theca interna. I.T. = Interstitial tissue. C.L. = Corpora lutea. G.E. = Germinal epithelium.

TABLE 10

Demonstration of 16β-Hydroxysteroid dehydrogenase in the ovary

Species	Substrate	Distribution	Investigators
Mouse	3β, 16β-Dihydroxyandrost-5-ene-3-methyl ether	a.G., T.I., I.T., C.L.	Baillie et al. (1966)
Rat	3β, 16β-Dihydroxyandrost-5-ene-3-methyl ether	a.G., T.I., I.T., C.L.	M. M. Ferguson (unpublished)
Mouse	16β-Hydroxyoestrone	a.G., T.I., I.T., C.L.	
	3β, 16β-Dihydroxyandrost-5-ene-3-methyl ether	a.G., T.I., I.T., C.L.	
Hamster	16β-Hydroxyoestrone	a.G., T.I., I.T., C.L.	
	3β, 16β-Dihydroxyandrost-5-ene-3-methyl ether	a.G., T.I., I.T.	
Guinea-pig	16β-Hydroxyoestrone	a.G., T.I., I.T.	
	3β, 16β-Dihydroxyandrost-5-ene-3-methyl ether	T.I., I.T., C.L.	
Rabbit	16β-Hydroxyoestrone	T.I., I.T., C.L.	
	3β, 16β-Dihydroxyandrost-5-ene-3-methyl ether	a.G., I.T., G.E.	
Cow	16β-Hydroxyoestrone	a.G., I.T., G.E.	
	3β, 16β-Dihydroxyandrost-5-ene-3-methyl ether	C.L.	
Sheep	16β-Hydroxyoestrone	C.L.	
	3β, 16β-Dihydroxyandrost-5-ene-3-methyl ether	C.L.	
Pig	16β-Hydroxyoestrone	C.L.	
	3β, 16β-Dihydroxyandrost-5-ene-3-methyl ether	T.I., I.T., C.L.	
Fowl	16β-Hydroxyoestrone	T.I., I.T., C.L.	
	3β, 16β-Dihydroxyandrost-5-ene-3-methyl ether	G., T.I.	
Frog	16β-Hydroxyoestrone	G., T.I.	
	3β, 16β-Dihydroxyandrost-5-ene-3-methyl ether	I.T.	
Human	16β-Hydroxyoestrone	I.T.	
	3β, 16β-Dihydroxyandrost-5-ene-3-methyl ether	a.G., T.I. C.L.	M. M. Ferguson and D. McK. Hart (unpublished)
Mouse (developing)	16β-Hydroxyoestrone	a.G., T.I. C.L.	
	3β, 16β-Dihydroxyandrost-5-ene-3-methyl ether	a.G., T.I., I.T., C.L., G.E.	Hart et al. (1966)

G. = Normal granulosa. a.G. = Atretic granulosa. T.I. = Theca interna.
I.T. = Interstitial tissue. C.L. = Corpora lutea. G.E. = Germinal epithelium.

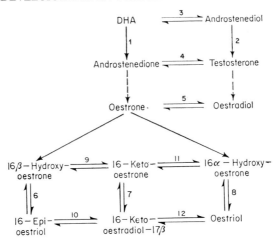

FIG. 53. Metabolic pathways of 16- and 17-hydroxysteroids. Reactions 1 and 2 are catalysed by 3β-hydroxysteroid dehydrogenase, reactions 3–8 by 17β-hydroxysteroid dehydrogenase, reactions 9 and 10 by 16β-hydroxysteroid dehydrogenase, and reactions 11 and 12 by 16α-hydroxysteroid dehydrogenase.

Although 16β-hydroxysteroid dehydrogenase is thought to be concerned with oestrogen metabolism (Fig. 54) (Breuer, 1959; Breuer *et al.*, 1959), a reaction of such intensity seems likely to be more significant than has hitherto been realised.

G. 17β-HYDROXYSTEROID DEHYDROGENASE

The distribution of 17β-hydroxysteroid dehydrogenase in the ovary recorded by various workers is summarized in Table 11.

Conflicting opinions exist on the histochemical distribution of 17β-hydroxysteroid dehydrogenase in the ovary. Wattenberg (1958), Pearson and Grose (1959b) and Goldberg *et al.* (1964) found no evidence of activity. Levy *et al.* (1959b) demonstrated weak activity in the same sites as 3β-hydroxysteroid dehydrogenase (i.e. *not* in germinal epithelium); and Ferguson (unpublished) noted an intense reaction in the germinal epithelium. The rat germinal epithelium uses a wide range of 17β-hydroxysteroids but only with NAD; NADP was not a suitable co-factor, as could have been foreseen from the poor NADP diaphorase in the germinal epithelium (Ferguson, unpublished).

Oestrone and oestradiol are well known to be secreted by the ovary (MacCorquodale *et al.*, 1936; Westerfield, *et al.*, 1938; Wotiz *et al.*, 1956; Smith, 1960; Short, 1962a; Gospodarowicz, 1964), as are testosterone (Kase *et al.*, 1961; Mahesh and Greenblatt, 1962; Depaoli and Eik-nes, 1963) and androstenediol, (Gospodarowicz, 1964). 17β-Hydroxysteroid dehydrogenase has also been demonstrated biochemically in ovary (Dowben and Rabinowitz,

TABLE 11

Demonstration of 17β-hydroxysteroid dehydrogenase in the ovary

Species	Substrate	Distribution	Investigators
Rabbit	Testosterone	Not demonstrated	Wattenberg (1958)
Human			
Rat	Oestradiol	Not demonstrated	Pearson and Grose (1959b)
Rat	Testosterone		
Rat	Testosterone	a.G., T.I., I.T., C.L.	Levy et al. (1959b)
Human	Testosterone and oestradiol	Not demonstrated	Fuhrmann (1961)
Dog			
Rat			
Human	3β, 17β-Dihydroxyandrostane	Not demonstrated	Goldberg et al. (1964)
	Testosterone, Nortestosterone		
	17β-Hydroxyandrosta-1,4-diene-3-one		
Rat	Oestradiol	G.E.	M. M. Ferguson (unpublished)
	Oestradiol	G.E.	
	Testosterone	G.E.	
	Oestradiol	G.E.	
Rabbit	Testosterone	I.T.	
	Oestradiol	I.T.	
Frog	Testosterone	I.T.	
	Oestrone	I.T.	
Fowl	Oestradiol	G., T.I.	
	Testosterone	G., T.I.	
Human	Oestradiol	C.L.	M. M. Ferguson (unpublished)
	Testosterone	C.L.	
Mouse (developing)	Oestradiol	G.E.	Hart et al. (1966)
	Testosterone	G.E.	
Rat	Nortestosterone	G.E.	M. M. Ferguson (unpublished)
	17β-Hydroxy-5α-androstan-3-one	G.E.	
	17β-Hydroxy-5β-androstan-3-one	G.E.	

G. = Normal granulosa. a.G. = Atretic granulosa. T.I. = Theca interna. I.T. = Interstitial tissue.
C.L. = Corpora lutea. G.E. = Germinal epithelium.

1956; Breuer, 1959; Breuer *et al.*, 1959), and its selective localization in the germinal epithelium in rodents is surprising and will be considered further below (p. 95).

H. 20α-HYDROXYSTEROID DEHYDROGENASE

The distribution of 20α-hydroxysteroid dehydrogenase in the ovary is shown in Table 12.

TABLE 12

Demonstration of 20α-hydroxysteroid dehydrogenase in the ovary

Species	Substrate	Distribution	Investigators
Rat	20α-Hydroxyprogesterone	C.L.	Balogh (1964); Balogh *et al.* (1966)
Rat	20α-Hydroxyprogesterone	C.L.	M. M. Ferguson (unpublished)

C. L. = Corpora lutea.

Histochemically in the rat 20α-hydroxysteroid dehydrogenase is NADP linked and is confined to the corpora lutea, with maximal activity seen during involution (Balogh, 1964). 20α-Hydroxyprogesterone, an active progestogen, is a progesterone metabolite secreted by the ovary (Zander, 1959; Wiest *et al.*, 1959; Wiest, 1963), and has been isolated from corpora lutea (Huang and Pearlman, 1962; Short, 1962a; Huang and Pearlman, 1963; Hammerstein *et al.*, 1964).

I. 20β-HYDROXYSTEROID DEHYDROGENASE

The distribution of 20β-hydroxysteroid dehydrogenase in the ovary is shown in Table 13.

TABLE 13

Demonstration of 20β-hydroxysteroid dehydrogenase in the ovary

Species	Substrate	Distribution	Investigators
Mouse	20β-Hydroxyprogesterone	T.I.	Baillie *et al.* (1965)

T.I. = Theca interna.

The reaction in the mouse ovary seen following incubation with 20β-hydroxyprogesterone was extremely weak and of doubtful significance.

20β-Hydroxyprogesterone, like 20α-hydroxyprogesterone, is an active progestin and has been isolated from bovine (Gorski *et al.*, 1958; Bowerman and Melampy, 1962), human (Zander, 1959) and whale ovaries (Kristoffersen *et al.*, 1961) and also from bovine follicular fluid (Short, 1962a, b). Moreover, Engel and Langer (1961) isolated 20α- and 20β-hydroxyprogesterone from bovine corpora lutea but only 20α-hydroxyprogesterone from rodent tissue, and this would explain the poor results obtained in mouse.

II. Tissues

A. FOLLICLE

Ova. The presence of *weak* 3α- and 16β-hydroxysteroid dehydrogenase in mouse ova is interesting (Fig. 54); normal follicles have no obvious activity, whereas some apparently atretic follicles occur with hydroxysteroid dehydrogenases either in the ovum alone or in the ovum and granulosa (Fig. 54).

Fig. 54. Mouse ovary incubated with 3α-hydroxy-5β-androstan-17-one, showing formazan deposited in ovum and granulosa of presumably atretic follicle. × 280.

Granulosa. Björkman (1962), in a study of the ultrastructure of the rat granulosa, describes a cellular architecture suggestive of protein secretion, which is in keeping with the concept that the granulosa cells secrete the liquor folliculi. On luteinization, which commences prior to ovulation in many species, including the rat, ultrastructural features characteristic of steroid secretion can be seen.

D

In the developing mouse ovary (Hart *et al.*, 1966a) between birth and three weeks, 3α-, Δ^5-3β- and 16β-hydroxysteroid dehydrogenase were seen in virtually all follicles, and the large number of histochemically active follicles is probably related to the high rate of follicular atresia at this time. After three weeks different patterns emerge in the mouse. The granulosa of some apparently normal follicles was histochemically inert; others, obviously atretic, had extensive formazan distributed throughout the membrana granulosa with activity distributed round the periphery of the cells. Finally, in many follicles some hydroxysteroid dehydrogenase activity was observed in the outer half of the membrana granulosa, whereas granulosa cells nearest the antral cavity were unreactive. This may represent the early stages of luteinization in pre-ovulatory and in atretic follicles. It would appear, from these histochemical findings, that the process of luteinization commences at the periphery of the membrana granulosa and spreads towards the antrum. Hydroxysteroid dehydrogenase activity in normal granulosa seems peculiar to the fowl ovary (Botte, 1963b; Wyburn and Baillie, 1964; Chieffi and Botte, 1965; M. M. Ferguson, unpublished).

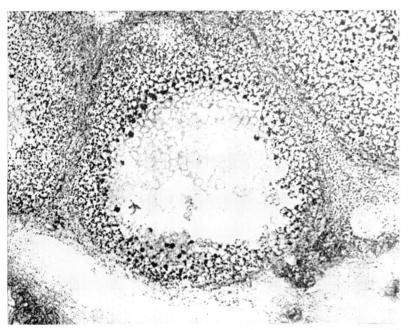

Fig. 55. Δ^5-3β-Hydroxysteroid dehydrogenase activity in $4\frac{1}{2}$-week-old mouse ovary. Note two distinct zones of granulosa. $\times 200$.

The liquor folliculi is known biochemically to contain numerous steroids (Short, 1961a, b; Short, 1962a, b; Lunaas, 1963), but their origin is not clear, although Short (1962a) considered that they are probably derived from the theca interna. The granulosa has also been implicated in a more complex relationship with the theca interna in which the theca interna is thought to be responsible for the biosynthesis of basic steroids and the granulosa for A-ring aromatization. Although this is in agreement with the observed histochemical restriction of Δ^5-3β-hydroxysteroid dehydrogenase (Fig. 55) to the theca interna of growing follicles, it must be borne in mind that the diaphorase content of normal granulosa is low, and this may be a limiting factor in the demonstration of hydroxysteroid dehydrogenases in granulosa.

Brambell (1956) has suggested three phases of liquor secretion: the first coincides with early antral formation, the second is pre-ovulatory and the third post-ovulatory. It may be that during the second phase of secretion luteinization commences in some granulosa cells, and this could account directly for the presence of some steroids in the liquor folliculi. It is possible that the fairly sizeable superficial pre-ovulatory follicles which have been the subject of biochemical investigation have commenced luteinization; this underlines the desirability of a joint histochemical and biochemical approach to studies of the granulosa.

Theca Interna. In the literature considerable confusion exists as to the precise status of the theca interna. Levy *et al.* (1959a, b) state that 3β-hydroxysteroid dehydrogenase is present in the theca interna, and that group of workers (Rubin *et al.*, 1963b) believes that activity increases with advancing maturity. The reverse view is held by Taylor (1961), who claims a diminution in intensity with age in rats.

In a recent review of ovarian steroidogenesis Ryan and Smith (1965) adduce evidence suggesting oestrogen biosynthesis from acetate in the Graafian follicle. The presence of 3α-, 3β-, 6β-, 11β-, 16α- and 16β-hydroxysteroid dehydrogenases in the theca interna (Tables 5–10) points to extensive steroid biosynthesis and metabolism in this tissue.

B. INTERSTITIAL TISSUE

The exact origin and significance of the ovarian interstitial tissue is not settled and there is considerable species variation in quantity: it is sparse in primates but relatively common in rodentia, lagomorpha and carnivora. Cyclical changes have been recorded in the interstitial tissue (Neal and Harrison, 1958) which suggest some form of secretory activity.

At birth the mouse ovary is largely composed of mesenchymal cells which do not resemble mature ovarian interstitial tissue (Hart *et al.*, 1966a) but 3α-, Δ^5-3β-, 11β- and 16β-hydroxysteroids are utilized at this stage, and activity can be seen in the interstitial mesenchyme (Fig. 56) throughout development. A dual origin for interstitial tissue in rats has been proposed (Dawson and McCabe, 1951; Rennels, 1951): a primary type supposedly develops from granulosa cell cords and occurs in immature animals and a secondary type is derived from the theca interna of atretic follicles. The recent histochemical findings with mouse ovary indicate differentiation of stromal mesenchymal cells into the 'primary type' of interstitial tissue with hydroxysteroid dehydrogenase activity evident at all stages of the transformation.

Interstitial cells with Δ^5-3β-hydroxysteroid dehydrogenase have been observed scattered throughout the human ovarian stroma (Ikonen *et al.*, 1961), and more recently Savard *et al.* (1965) presented biochemical evidence for the presence of this enzyme in the interstitial cells of the human ovary. It can therefore be concluded that the ovarian interstitial tissue serves some

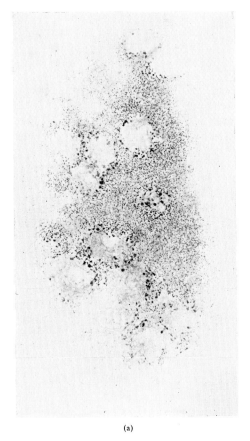

(a)

FIG. 56. (a) 3β-Hydroxysteroid dehydrogenase in neonatal mouse ovary showing unorganized reactive interstitial tissue. $\times$ 200.

steroidogenic function, and in our view this tissue constitutes another major site of ovarian steroid biosynthesis.

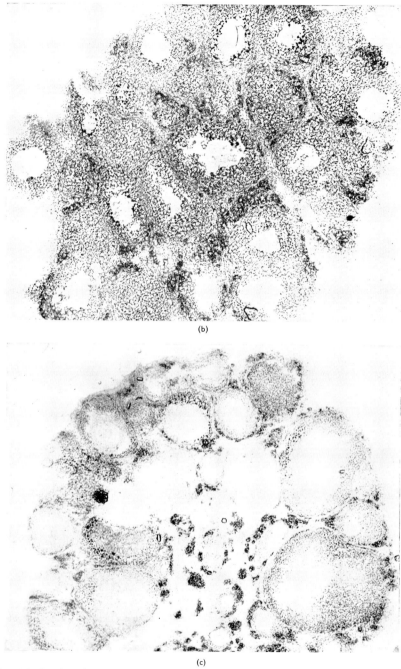

(b)

(c)

FIG. 56. Continued. (b) 2-Week-old mouse ovary showing activity with DHA. ×170.
(c) Further organization of 3β-hydroxysteroid dehydrogenase containing interstitial tissue in
the 4-week postnatal mouse ovary. ×130.

C. CORPORA LUTEA

Corpora lutea appear to be divided into at least two categories on a comparative biochemical basis; the first synthesizes only progestins, and the second is capable of the formation of multiple steroids including oestrogens (Savard, Marsh and Rice, 1965). Examples of the first group include cow and mare and the second group human and rat. Nevertheless, regardless of its category the corpus luteum can be expected to have histochemically demonstrable Δ^5-3β-hydroxysteroid dehydrogenase.

Wattenberg (1958) was able to demonstrate Δ^5-3β-hydroxysteroid dehydrogenase in rat and human corpora lutea but not in the rabbit. Rubin et al. (1963a) could only show weak activity in the theca lutein cells of the rabbit, but human, rat, mouse, guinea-pig, sheep, cow, horse and cat corpora lutea were all reactive. This condition in the rabbit corpus luteum is perplexing, as the blood concentration of progesterone in the oestrous cycle and pregnancy is thought to be dependent on the presence of a corpus luteum in the initial stages at least (Telegdy et al., 1963); but there may be some hitherto unexplained relationship between the corpus luteum and highly active interstitial tissue in the rabbit.

The pattern of 3α-, Δ^5-3β-, 6β-, 11β-, 16α-, 16β- and 20α-hydroxysteroid dehydrogenase activity in corpora lutea is similar in that from ovulation to the vascular phase there is an increase in enzymic activity which declines on

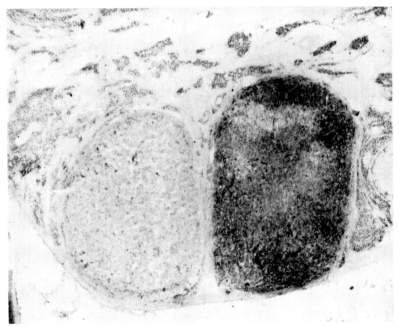

FIG. 57. Two corpora lutea of rat ovary incubated with pregnenolone, showing a marked difference in enzyme activity. × 80.

regression of the corpus luteum. Rat and mouse corpora lutea of previous cycles are usually active but much less intense (Fig. 57).

Ferguson (unpublished) has noted the appearance of a 3α-hydroxysteroid dehydrogenase in rat corpora lutea (Fig. 50) which is stereo-specific for androsterone. The corresponding 3α-hydroxy-5α-isomer is poorly utilized by the rat corpus luteum. Both androsterone and aetiocholanolone give a poor histochemical reaction in other ovarian tissues, including the theca interna and interstitial tissue. It is interesting to note that androsterone has been isolated biochemically from the corpus luteum (Simmer and Voss, 1960) and that the ovary has long been known to secrete androgens (Lipschutz, 1937; Parkes, 1937; Hill, 1950; Short, 1960). The production of androsterone by the corpus luteum could be associated with the inhibition of ovulation, but this possibility is speculative. Other metabolic possibilities, supported by biochemical precedent, are indicated in Fig. 58.

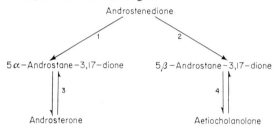

FIG. 58. Metabolism of 3α-hydroxysteroids. Reactions 1 and 2 are catalysed by Δ^5 reductases, and reactions 3 and 4 by 3α-hydroxysteroid dehydrogenase.

If corpus luteal 3α-hydroxysteroid dehydrogenase is concerned in the formation of androsterone or the corresponding pregnane derivative, then the possibility exists that this enzyme has a dual function, in view of its supposed transhydrogenase function referred to above.

In conclusion, it seems reasonable to regard the corpus luteum as another principal site of ovarian androgen, oestrogen and progestogen (for example, 20α- and 20β-hydroxyprogesterone) biosynthesis.

In a sense the biochemical activities of the corpus luteum are better understood than those of the other two principal steroid biosynthetic sites, but much remains to be done to integrate fully the observed presence of enzymes such as 16β-hydroxysteroid dehydrogenase with its function in maintaining pregnancy.

D. THE GERMINAL EPITHELIUM

Steroid biosynthesis is not associated with the germinal epithelium, and this is in keeping with its lack of demonstrable Δ^5-3β-hydroxysteroid dehydrogenase. Some workers have proposed that its mitotic activity at oestrus is due to oestrogenic stimulation (Stein and Allen, 1942; Bullough, 1946), although others (Zuckerman, 1951; Harrison, 1962) attribute this to general ovarian enlargement.

It is difficult to relate these facts to the specific and striking 17β-hydroxy-steroid dehydrogenase present in mouse (Hart *et al.*, 1966) rabbit and rat, (M. M. Ferguson, unpublished) germinal epithelium (Fig. 59). This enzyme, together with the weak 16α- and 16β-hydroxysteroid dehydrogenase present in the germinal epithelium, would seem to be concerned with the metabolism of 16- and 17- hydroxysteroids, presumably oestrogenic in nature.

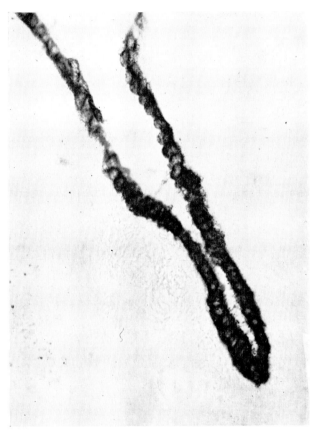

FIG. 59. 17β-Hydroxysteroid dehydrogenase activity confined to geminal epithelium of rat ovary with testosterone as substrate. $\times 250$.

E. OVARIAN TUMOURS

This interesting field of histochemistry is, at the time of writing, largely virgin territory. Acosta (1962) and Goldberg *et al.* (1963b) seem to be the only workers so far involved in this field, and weak 3β-hydroxysteroid dehydrogenase was noted in an androgen-secreting arrhenoblastoma and in a progesterone-producing luteinized granulosa cell tumour.

REFERENCES

Acosta, A. (1962). Microscopic histochemistry investigation of steroid 3β-ol dehydrogenase in Stein-Leventhal type of ovaries. Thesis, University of Cordoba, Argentina. (Quoted by Goldberg *et al.*, 1963).

Baillie, A. H., Calman, K. C., Ferguson, M. M. and Hart, D. McK. (1965). Histochemical demonstration of 20β-hydroxysteroid dehydrogenase. *J. Endocrinol.* **32**, 337–339.

Baillie, A. H., Calman, K. C., Ferguson, M. M. and Hart, D. McK. (1966). Histochemical utilization of 3α-, 6β-, 11α-, 12α-, 16α-, 16β-, 17α-, 21- and 24-hydroxysteroids. *J. Endocrinol.* **34**, 1–12.

Baillie, A. H., Ferguson, M. M., Calman, K. C. and Hart, D. McK. (1965). Histochemical demonstration of 11β-hydroxysteroid dehydrogenase. *J. Endocrinol.* **33**, 119–125.

Balogh, K. (1964). A histochemical method for the demonstration of 20α-hydroxysteroid dehydrogenase activity in rat ovaries. *J. Histochem. Cytochem.* **12**, 670–673.

Balogh, K., Kidwell, W. R. and Wiest, W. G. (1966). Histochemical localization of rat ovarian 20α-hydroxysteroid dehydrogenase activity initiated by G. H. administration. *Endocrinology* **78**, 75–81.

Bara, G. (1965). Histochemical localization of Δ⁵-3β-hydroxysteroid dehydrogenase in the ovaries of a teleost fish, Scamber Scamber L. Gen. Comp. Endocrin. **5**, 284–296.

Baron, D. N., Gare, M. B. R., Pietruszko, R. and Williams, D. C. (1963). Purification and properties of the 3α-hydroxysteroid-dependent nicotinamide-adenine dinucleotide transhydrogenase of rat liver. *Biochem. J.* **88**, 19–25.

Björkman, N. (1962). A study of the ultrastructure of the granulosa cells of the rat ovary. *Acta Anat.* **51**, 125–147.

Bloch, E., Romney, S. L., Klein, M., Lipiello, L., Cooper, P. and Goldring, I. P. (1965). Steroid synthesis by human fetal adrenals and ovaries maintained in organic culture. *Proc. Soc. Exptl. Biol. Med.* **119**, 449–452.

Botte, V (1963a). Histochemical and histological investigations of the post-ogulatory and atretic follicles of Raja sp. *Acta Med. Romana* **1**, 1–7.

Botte, V. (1963b). La localizzazione della steroide-3β-olo-deidrogenasi nell' ovaio di pollo. *Rend. 1st. Sci. Univ. Camerino* **4**, 205–209.

Botte, V. and Del Bianco, C. (1962). "Research in the histochemical distribution of lipids and steroid-3β-ol-dehydrogenase in the ovaries of immature rats treated with gonadotropins." *Arch. Ostet. Ginecol.* **67**, 653–665.

Bowerman A. M. and Melampy, R. M. (1962). Progesterone and Δ⁴-pregnen-20-ol-3-one in bovine reproductive organs and body fluids. *Proc. Soc. Exptl. Biol. Med.* **109**, 48–48.

Brambell, F. W. R. (1956). In: *Marshall's Physiology of Reproduction* Vol. 1. (Longmans, Green, London).

Breuer, H. (1959). Recent results in the field of oestrogen metabolism. *Arzneimittel-Forsch.* **9**, 667–671.

Breuer, H., Knuppen, R. and Pangels, G. (1959). Stoffwechsel von 16-Ketooestron in Menschlichen Geweben endocriner Organe. *Acta Endocrinol.* **30**, 247–258.

Bullough, W. S. (1946). Mitotic activity in the adult mouse, Mus musculus L. A study of its relation to the oestrous cycle in normal and abnormal conditions. *Phil. Trans. Roy. Soc. London, Ser. B* **231**, 453–516.

Chang, E. and Dao, T. L. (1962). Adrenal oestrogens. II. Further characterizations of isolated urinary 11β-hydroxysterone and 11β-hydroxyestradiol. *Biochim. Biophys. Acta.* **57**, 609–612.

Chieffi, G. (1962). Endocrine aspects of reproduction in elasmobranch fishes. *Gen. Comp. Endocrinol., Suppl.* **1**, 275–285.

Chieffi, G. and Botte, V. (1963). Osservazioni istochimiche sull' attivita della steroide-3β-olo-deidrogenasi nell interrenole e nelle gonadi di girini e adulti Rana esculenta. *Atti del IV Congresso Nazionale della Societa Italiana di Istochimica.*

Chieffi, G. and Botte, V. (1965). The distribution of some enzymes involved in the steroidogenesis of hens ovary. *Experientia* **21**, 16–17.

Claesson, L. (1954). Quantitative relationship between gonadotrophic stimulation and lipid changes in the interstitial gland of the rabbit ovary. *Acta Physiol. Scand. Suppl.* **113**, 23–51.

Claesson, L. and Hillarp, N. A. (1947a). The formation mechanism of oestrogenic hormones. I. *Acta Physiol. Scand.* **13**, 115–129.

Claesson, L. and Hillarp, N. A. (1947b). The formation mechanism of oestrogenic hormones II. *Acta Physiol. Scand.* **14**, 102–119.

Cohn, G. L. and Mulrow, P. J. (1961). *Proc. Endocrine Soc., 43rd Meeting, N.Y.* p. 52.

Dawson, A. B. and McCabe, M. (1951). The interstitial tissue of the ovary in infantile and juvenile rats. *J. Morphol.* **88**, 543–571.

Deane, H. W. (1952). Histochemical observations on the ovary and oviduct of the albino rat during the estrous cycle. *Am. J. Anat.* **91**, 363–413.

Deane, H. W., Lobel, B. L., Driks, E. C. and Rubin, B. L. (1961). Further observations on steroid-3β-ol dehydrogenase activity in the reproductive system of the female rat. *Am. Histochem.* **6**, 283–291.

Deane, H. W., Lobel, B. L. and Romney, S. L. (1962). Enzymic histochemistry of normal human ovaries of the menstrual cycle, pregnancy and the early puerperium. *Am. J. Obstet. Gynecol.* **83**, 281–294

Deane, H. W. and Rubin, B. L. (1965). Identification and control of cells that synthesize steroid hormones in the adrenal glands, gonads and placentae of various mammalian species. *Arch. Anat. Microscop. Morphol. Exp.* **54**, 49–65.

Dempsey, E. W. and Bassett, D. L. (1943). Observations on the fluorescence, birefringence and histochemistry of the rat ovary during the reproductive cycle. *Endocrinology* **33**, 384–401.

Depaoli, J. and Eik-Nes, K. B. (1963). Metabolism *in vivo* of (7α-^{3}H) pregnenolone by the dog ovary. *Biochim. Biophys. Acta.* **78**, 457–465.

Diczfalusy, E., Cassmer, O., Alonso, C. and De Miquel, M. (1961). Oestrogen metabolism in the human foetus. II. Oestrogen conjugation by foetal organs *in vitro* and *in vivo*. *Acta Endocrinol.* **37**, 516–528.

Dowben, R. M. and Rabinowitz, J. L. (1956). Oxidation *in vitro* of radioactive oestradiol by preparations of human tissue. *Nature* **178**, 696.

Engel, L. L. and Langer, L. J. (1961). Biochemistry of steroid hormones. *Ann. Rev. Biochem.* **30**, 499–425.

Everett, J. W. (1947). Hormonal factors responsible for deposition of cholesterol in the corpus luteum of the rat. *Endocrinology* **41**, 364–377.

Ferguson, M. M. (1965). 3β-Hydroxysteroid dehydrogenase activity in the mouse ovary. *J. Endocrinol.* **32**, 365–371.

Fienberg, R. and Cohen, R. B. (1965). A comparative histochemical study of the ovarian stromal lipid, stromal theca cell, and nomal ovarian follicular apparatus. *Am. J. Obstet. Gynecol.* **92**, 958–969.

Forleo, Rand Collins, W. P. (1964). Some aspects of Steroid biosynthesis in human ovarian tissue. *Acta Endocrinol.* **46**, 265–278.

Fuhrmann, K. (1961). Uber den histochemischen Nachweis der 3β-ol-Steroiddehydrogenase-Aktivitat in Geweben endokriner Organe. *Zentr. Gynaekol.* **83**, 565–572.

Fuhrmann, K. (1963), Histochemische Untersuchungen uber Hydroxysteroid Dehydrogenase-Aktivitat in Nebennieren und Eierstocken von Ratten und Kaninchen. *Arch Gynaekol.* **197**, 583–600.

Goldberg, B., Jones, G. E. S. and Borkowf, H. I. (1964). A histochemical study of substrate specificity for the steroid 3β-ol dehydrogenase and isomerase systems in human ovary and testes. *J. Histochem. Cytochem.* **12**, 880–889.

Goldberg, B., Jones, G. E. and Turner, D. A. (1963). Steroid-3β-ol dehydrogenase activity in human endocrine tissues. *Am. J. Obstet. Gynecol.* **86**, 349–359.

Goldberg, B., Jones, G. E. and Woodruff, J. D. (1963b). A histochemical study of steroid 3β-ol dehydrogenase activity in some steroid producing tumours. *Am. J. Obstet. Gynecol.* **86**, 1003–1014.

Goldman, A. S., Yakovac, W. C. and Bongiovanni, A. M. (1966). Development of activity of 3β-hydroxysteroid dehydrogenase in human fetal tissues and in two anencephalic newborns *J. Clin. Endocrinol. Metab.* **26**, 14–22.

Goldman, A. S., Yakovac, W. C. and Bongiovanni, A. M. (1965). Persistent effects of a synthetic androstene derivative on activities of 3β-hydroxysteroid dehydrogenase and glucose-6-phosphate dehydrogenase in rats. *Endocrinology* **77**, 1105–1118.

Gorski, J., Dominiguez, O. V., Samuels, L. T. and Erb, R. E. (1958). Progestins of the bovine ovary. *Endocrinology* **62**, 234–235.

Gospodarowicz, D. (1964). The action of follicle stimulating hormone and of human chorionic gonadotrophin upon steroid synthesis by rabbit ovarian tissues *in vitro*. *Acta Endocrinol.* **47**, 293–305.

Hammerstein, J., Rice, B. F. and Savard, K. (1964). Steroid hormone formation in the human ovary: I. Identification of steroids formed *in vitro* from acetate-1-^{14}C in the corpus luteum. *J. Clin. Endocrinol. Metab.* **24**, 597–605.

Harrison, R. J. (1962). In: *The Ovary* (Ed. Zuckerman), Ch. 2C (Academic Press, New York).

Hart, D. McK., Baillie, A. H., Calman, K. C. and Ferguson, M. M. (1966a). Hydroxysteroid dehydrogenase development in the mouse adrenal and gonads. *J. Anat.* (in press).

Hart, D. McK., Calman, K. C., Ferguson, M. M., Niemi, M. and Baillie, A. H. (1966b). Hydroxysteroid dehydrogenase activity in human foetal gonads. Hart, M.D. Thesis. Glasgow University.

Hill, R. T. (1950). Multiplicity of ovarian functions in the mouse. *Arch. Anat. Microscop. Morphol. Exp.* **39**, 634–644.

Huang, W. Y. and Pearlman, W. H. (1962). The corpus luteum and steroid hormone formation. I. Studies on luteinized rat ovarian tissue *in vitro*. *J. Biol. Chem* **237**, 1060–1065.

Huang, W. Y. and Pearlman, W. H. (1963). The corpus luteum and steroid hormone formation. II. Studies on the human corpus luteum *in vitro*. *J. Biol. Chem.* **238**, 1308–1315.

Ikonen, M., Niemi, M., Personen, S. and Timonen, S. (1961). Histochemical localization of four dehydrogenase systems in the human ovary during the menstrual cycle. *Acta Endocrinol.* **38**, 293–302.

Kern-Bontke, E. (1964). Histochemisch Nachweisbare fermentaktivität in den Theca und Granulosaluteinzellen des Corpus Luteum. *Histochemie* **4**, 56–64.

Knuppen, R. and Breuer, H. (1962). Biogenesis of 11β-hydroxyoestrone and 16β-hydroxyoestrone by adrenal tissue. *Biochim. Biophys. Acta.* **58**, 147–148.

Koerner, D. R. and Hellman, L. (1964). Effect of thyroxine administration on the 11β-hydroxysteroid dehydrogenases in rat liver and kidney. *Endocrinology* **75**, 592–601.

Kristoffersen, J., Lunaas, T. and Velle, W. (1961). Identification of 20β-hydroxy-pregn-4-ene-3-one in luteal tissue from pregnant whales. *Nature* **190**, 1009–1010.

Kase, N., Forchielli, E. and Dorfman, R. I. (1961). *In vitro* production of testosterone and androst-4-ene-3, 17-dione in a human ovarian homogenate. *Acta Endocrinol.* **37**, 19–23.

Layne, D. S. and Marrian, G. F. (1958). The isolation of 16β-hydroxyoestrone and 16-oxo-oestradiol-17β from the urine of pregnant women. *Biochem. J.* **70**, 244–248.

Levy, H., Deane, H. W. and Rubin, B. L. (1959a). Observations on steroid 3β-ol dehydrogenase activity in steroid producing glands. *J. Histochem. Cytochem.* **7**, 320.

Levy, H., Deane, H. W. and Rubin, B. L. (1959b). Visualisation of steroid-3β-ol dehydrogenase activity in tissues of intact hypophysectomized rats. *Endocrinology* **65**, 932–943.

Lipschutz, A. (1937). Androgenic endocrine activity in the female-mammal. *Nature* **140**, 892.

Lunaas, T. (1963). Distribution of oestrone and oestradiol-17β in sow ovaries. *Acta Endocrinol.* **44**, 529–535.

McCorquodale, D. W., Thayer, S. A. and Doisy, E. A. (1936). The isolation of principal estrogenic substance of liquor folliculi. *J. Biol. Chem.* **115**, 435–448.

McKay, D. G. and Robinson, D. (1947). Observations on the fluorescence, birefringence and histochemistry of the human ovary during the menstrual cycle. *Endocrinology* **41**, 378–394.

Mahesh, V. B. and Greenblatt, R. B. (1962). Isolation of dehydroepiandrosterone and 17α-hydroxy-Δ^5-pregnenolone from the polycystic ovaries of the Stein-Leventhal Syndrome. *J. Clin. Endocrinol.* **22**, 441–448.

Narbaitz, R. and Kolodny, L. (1964). Δ^5-3β-OH-steroid dehydrogenase in differentiating chick gonads. *Z. Zellforsch. Mikroskop. Anat.* **63**, 612–617.

Neal, E. G. and Harrison, R. J. (1958). Reproduction in the European badger (Meles meles L.) *Trans. Zool. Soc. London* **29**, 67–131.

Noall, M. W., Alexander, F. and Allen, W. M. (1962). Dehydroisoandrosterone synthesis by the human ovary. *Biochim. Biophys. Acta.* **59**, 520–521.

Parkes, A. S. (1937). Androgenic activity of ovarian extracts. *Nature* **139**, 965.

Pearson, B. and Grose, F. (1959a). Histochemical study of some DPNH and DPN dependent dehydrogenases. *Federation Proc.* **18**, 499.

Pearson, B. and Grose, F. (1959b). Histochemical demonstration of 17β-hydroxysteroid dehydrogenase by use of a tetrazolium salt. *Proc. Soc. Exptl. Biol. Med.* **100**, 636–638.

Presl, J., Jirasek, J., Horsky, J. and Henzl, M. (1965). Observations on steroid 3β-ol dehydrogenase activity in the ovary during early postnatal development in the rat. *J. Endocrinol.* **31**, 293–294.

Price, D. and Pannabecker, R. (1956). Organ culture studies of foetal rat reproductive tracts. Ciba Found. Colloq. Aging **2**, 3–13.

Price, D., Ortiz, E. and Deane, H. W. (1964). The presence of a Δ^5-3β-hydroxysteroid dehydrogenase in fetal guinea-pig testis and adrenal glands. *Am. Zool.* **4**, No. 4.

Rennels, E. G. (1951). Influence of hormones on the histochemistry of ovarian interstitial tissue in the immature rat. *Am. J. Anat.* **88**, 63–108.

Roberts, J. D. and Warren, J. C. (1964). Steroid biosynthesis in the fetal ovary. *Endocrinology* **74**, 846–852.

Rubin, B. L. and Deane, H. W. (1965). Effects of superovulation on ovarian Δ^5-3β-hydroxysteroid dehydrogenase activity in rats of different ages. *Endocrinology* **76**, 382–389.

Rubin, B. L., Deane, H. W., Hamilton, J. A. and Driks, E. C. (1963a). Changes in Δ^5-3β-hydroxysteroid dehydrogenase activity in the ovaries of maturing rats. *Endocrinology* **72**, 924–930

Rubin, B. L., Deane, H. W. and Hamilton, J. A. (1963b). Biochemical and histochemical studies on Δ^5-3β-hydroxysteroid dehydrogenase activity in the adrenal glands and ovaries of diverse mammals. *Endocrinology* **73**, 748–763.

Rubin, B. L., Hamilton, J. A., Karlson, J. J. and Tufaro, R. I. (1965). Effect of the age of the rat at the time of hemicastration on the weight, estimated secretory activity and Δ^5-3β-hydroxysteroid dehydrogenase activity of the remaining ovary. *Endocrinology* **77**, 909–916.

Ryan, K. J. and Smith, O. W. (1961a). Biogenesis of estrogens by the human ovary. I. Conversion of acetate-1-C^{14} to estrone and estradiol. *J. Biol. Chem.* **236**, 705–709.

Ryan, K. J. and Smith, O. W (1961b) Biogenesis of estrogens by the human ovary. II. Conversion of progesterone-4-C^{14} to estrone and estradiol. *J. Biol. Chem.* **236**, 710–714.

Ryan, K. J. and Smith, O. W. (1961c). Biogenesis of estrogens by the human ovary. III. Conversion of cholesterol-4-C^{14} to estrone. *J. Biol. Chem.* **236**, 2204–2206.

Ryan, K. J. and Smith, O. W. (1961d). Biogenesis of estrogens by the human ovary. IV. Formation of neutral steroid intermediates. *J. Biol. Chem.* **236**, 2207–2212.

Ryan, K. J. and Smith, O. W. (1965). Biogenesis of steroid hormones in the human. ovary. *Recent Progr. Hormone Res.* **21**, 367–403.

Savard, K., Gut, M., Dorfman, R. I., Gabrilove, J. L. and Soffer, L. J. (1961). Formation of human androgens by human arrhenoblastoma tissue *in vitro*. *J. Clin. Endocrinol.* **21**, 165.

Savard, K., Marsh, J. M. and Rice, B. F. (1965). Gonadotropins and ovarian steroidogenesis. *Recent Progr. Hormone Res.* **21**, 285–356.

Short, R. V. (1960). Steroids present in the follicular fluid of the mare. *J. Endocrinol.* **20**, 147–156.

Short, R. V. (1961a). Δ^5-3β-hydroxysteroids in the follicular fluid of the mare. *J. Endocrinol* **23**, 277–283.

Short, R. V. (1961b). Steroid concentrations in the follicular fluid of mares at various stages of the reproductive cycle. *J. Endocrinol.* **22**, 153–163.

Short, R. V. (1962a). Steroids in the follicular fluid and the corpus luteum of the mare. A "two-cell type" theory of ovarian steroid synthesis. *J. Endocrinol* **24**, 59–63.

Short, R. V. (1962b). Steroid concentrations in normal follicular fluid and ovarian cyst fluid from cows. *J. Reprod. Fertility* **4**, 27–45.

Short, R. V. (1964). Ovarian steroid synthesis and secretion in vivo. *Recent Progr. Hormone Res.* **20**, 303-333.

Simmer, H. and Voss, H. A. (1960). Androgens in the human ovary. *Klin. Wochschr.* **38**, 819–822.

Smith, O. W. (1960). Estrogens in ovarian fluids of normally menstruating women. *Endocrinology* **67**, 698–707.

Stein, K. F. and Allen, E. (1942). Attempts to stimulate proliferation of the germinal epithelium of the ovary. *Anat. Record* **83**, 193–207.

Talalay, P. (1957). Enzymatic mechanism in steroid metabolism. *Physiol. Rev.* **37**, 362–389.

Tamaoki, B. I. and Pincus, G. (1961). Biogenesis of progesterone in ovarian tissues. *Endocrinology* **69**, 527–533.

Taylor, F. B. (1961). Histochemical changes in ovaries of normal and experimentally treated rats. *Acta Endocrinol.* **36**, 361–374.

Telegdy, G., Endoczi, E. and Lissak, K. (1963). Ovarian progesterone secretion during the oestrous cycle, pregnancy and lactation in dogs. *Acta Endocrinol.* **44**, 461–466.

Tomkins, G. M. (1956). A mammalian 3β-hydroxysteroid dehydrogenase. *J. Biol. Chem.* **218**, 437–447.

Turolla, E. and Magrini, U. (1963). Attivita 3 beta-idrossi-steroide deidrogenasiia e glucoso-6-fosfato deidrogenasiia nell ovaia di ratta normale. *Folia Endocrinol. (Pisa)* **16**, 474–483.

Varangot, J. and Cedard, L. (1962). Determination of serum oestrogens during normal pregnancy. *Bull. Federation Soc. Gynecol. Obstet. Langue Franc.* **13**, 371–373.

Warren, J. C. and Salhanick, H. A. (1961). Steroid biosynthesis in the human ovary. *J. Clin. Endocrinol.* **21**, 1218–1230.

Wattenberg, L. W. (1958). Microscopic histochemical demonstration of steroid-3β-ol dehydrogenase in tissue sections. *J. Histochem. Cytochem.* **6**, 225–232.

Westerfield, W. W., McCorquodale, D. W., Thayer, S. A. and Doisy, E. A. (1938). The isolation of Theelin from human placenta. *J. Biol. Chem.* **126**, 195–200.

Wiest, W. G. (1963). *In vitro* metabolism of progesterone and 20-hydroxy-pregn-4-en-3-one by tissues of the female rat. *Endocrinology* **73**, 310–316.

Wiest, W. G., Zander, J. and Holmstrom, E. G. (1959). Metabolism of progesterone-4-C¹⁴ by an arrhenoblastoma. *J. Clin. Endocrinol Metab.* **19**, 297–305.

Wotiz, H. H. and Davis, J. W., Lemon, H. M. and Gut, M. (1956). Studies in steroid metabolism. V. The conversion of testosterone-4-C¹⁴ to estrogens by human ovarian tissue. *J. Biol. Chem.* **216**, 677.

Wyburn, G. M. and Baillie, A. H. (1964). Some observations on the fine structure and histochemistry of the ovarian follicle of the fowl. British Egg Marketing Board.

Zander, J. (1959). In: *Recent Progress in the Endocrinology of Reproduction* (Ed. Lloyd) (Academic Press, New York).

Zuckerman, S. (1951). The number of oöcytes in the mature ovary. *Recent Progr. Hormone Res.* **6**, 63–109.

CHAPTER 6

The Adrenal Cortex

The adrenal cortex has attracted investigators in every branch of biology. The three major zones, defined by Arnold (1866) and confirmed by Gottschau (1883), tended to be considered functionally separate until relatively recently. In this chapter the species and zonal distribution of indvidual hydroxysteroid dehydrogenases will be detailed and an attempt will then be made to relate these findings to current views on functional adrenal zonation.

I. 3α-HYDROXYSTEROID DEHYDROGENASE

This enzyme is not convincing as a histochemical entity in most adrenals studied. It is absent from frog adrenal glands, and Pearson and Grose (1959a) failed to demonstrate it in rat adrenal. Baillie *et al.* (1966) and Hart *et al.* (1966) noted trace 3α-hydroxysteroid dehydrogenase activity in all zones of rat and mouse adrenal cortices, respectively. In the adult human adrenal cortex, weak 3α-hydroxysteroid dehydrogenase activity (Calman *et al.*, 1966) is demonstrable in the outer part of the zona fasciculata and, perhaps, in the zona reticularis. The weak nature of these positive reactions, however, must be stressed; traces of pink monoformazan only are deposited. By contrast, recent work in this laboratory indicates the presence of moderate 3α-hydroxysteroid dehydrogenase activity in the hamster adrenal.

In the foetal human adrenal gland the situation is rather different: although the definitive cortex is almost unreactive (Calman *et al.*, 1966), moderate 3α-hydroxysteroid dehydrogenase activity is present with either 5α- or 5β-steroids in the foetal zone. Similarly, in the developing mouse adrenal 3α-hydroxysteroid dehydrogenase can be located histochemically in the cortex of embryos aged 17 days and over (Hart *et al.*, 1966). The reaction is strongest in the zona fasciculata and diminishes rapidly after birth. It was tentatively suggested by Calman *et al.* (1966) that the presence of 3α-hydroxysteroid dehydrogenase in the foetal adrenal might be related to the detoxication of steroids, perhaps of maternal origin.

II. Δ⁵-3β-HYDROXYSTEROID DEHYDROGENASE

There is no doubt that this enzyme can be demonstrated histochemically in all normal adrenal cortices (Table 14), but, particularly in the human adrenal, detail differences occur with regard to its zonal distribution as reported by different workers. To summarize, in the adult human adrenal 3β-hydroxy-

TABLE 14

Demonstration of Δ^5 -3β-hydroxysteroid dehydrogenase in the adrenal gland

Species	Substrate	Observations	Investigator
Human, rat, rabbit, mouse	Pregnenolone and DHA	In all species all (cortical) cells are positive but the reaction in the zona glomerulosa is weak	Wattenberg (1958)
Rat	DHA	All zones exhibit 3β-hydroxysteroid dehydrogenase activity	Levy et al. (1959)
Human	DHA	All zones show some activity but the fascicular reaction is strongest	Cavallero and Chiappino (1961)
Human and rat	Pregnenolone and DHA	All zones show some activity but the fascicular reaction is strongest	Dawson et al. (1961a)
Human adult	DHA	Moderate reaction in zona glomerulosa; heavy staining in outer fasciculata; little reaction in the inner fasciculata and reticularis	Dawson et al. (1961b)
Human foetal	DHA	Activity appears at 11 weeks in the foetal and definitive cortices	
Rat	DHA	All zones reactive	
Rabbit and rat	Pregnenolone and DHA	All zones are reactive	Fuhrmann (1961)
Chrysemis sp. Varanus niloticus L. Natrix natrix L. Gallus gallus Perdix perdix Coturnix coturnix Alectoris rufa L. Phasianus colchicus L.	DHA	Activity is less marked in the peripheral zone of the cortex	Arvy (1962)
Human foetal	DHA	Activity in both foetal and definitive cortex	Bloch et al. (1962)
Human	DHA	Outer (clear) cells strongly positive; remainder weak	Cavallero and Chiappino (1962)
Rabbit and rat	Pregnenolone and DHA	All zones are reactive	Fuhrmann (1963)
Human	DHA	All zones are active, except the inner part of the zona fasciculata	Goldberg et al. (1963)
Rat	DHA	All zones reactive; activity increases in zona glomerulosa if sodium intake is restricted or angiotensin given	Marx and Deane (1963)
Rat	DHA	All zones reactive; activity increases in zona glomerulosa if sodium intake is restricted or angiotensin given	Marx et al. (1963)
Foetal armadillo	DHA	Reticular pattern of activity within the foetal cortex	Rubin et al. (1963)
Armadillo, cat, dog, guinea-pig, mouse, ox, rabbit and rat	DHA	All adrenocortical cells are active; no zonal differences were seen in the cat; the zona glomerulosa was markedly less reactive than the other two zones in armadillo, dog, mouse, ox, rabbit or rat	
Human	Pregnenolone 17α-hydroxy-pregnenolone DHA	Δ^5-3β-hydroxysteroid dehydrogenase not demonstrable in subjects excreting large amounts of Δ^5-3β-hydroxysteroids. Outer fascicular zone is heavily reactive; glomerulosa, inner fasciculata and reticularis are less reactive	Goldman et al. (1964)
Chicken	DHA	Adrenal active prior to hatching	Narbaitz and Kolodny (1964)
Mouse	Androstan-3β-ol-17-one (configuration not specified)	All zones reactive	Pearson et al. (1964)
Guinea-pig	DHA	All zones reactive	Price et al. (1964)
Human, monkey	Pregnenolone, 17α-hydroxy-pregnenolone, DHA, androstenediol	1. All substrates give a strong reaction in the outer part of the zona fasciculata, none in the inner part and a very poor reaction in the zona glomerulosa and zona reticularis	Baillie et al. (1965)
	Pregnenolone sulphate, 17α-hydroxypregnenolone sulphate, DHA sulphate	2. The first two sulphates give the same reaction as the corresponding free steroids; DHA sulphate was not used to any extent	
	Pregnenolone acetate, DHA acetate, 16α-hydroxy-pregnenolone	3. These steroids give the same histochemical pattern as the first four substrates listed (1)	

TABLE 14. Continued

Species	Substrate	Observations	Investigator
Human	DHA	Activity not demonstrated in adrenals of foetuses up to 28 cm	Cavallero et al. (1965)
Rat	DHA	Activity in all zones, weakest in zone reticularis	Freses et al. (1965)
Rat	Pregnenolone, 17α-hydroxy-pregnenolone, DHA	All zones reactive	Goldman et al. (1965)
Human foetal	Pregnenolone, 17α-hydroxy-pregnenolone, DHA, androstenediol	1. All steroids in this group were used by the foetal cortex; the definitive cortex was divided into an outer, unreactive zone and an inner reactive zone	Niemi and Baillie (1965)
	Pregnenolone sulphate, 17α-hydroxypregnenolone sulphate, DHA sulphate 3β-hydroxy-5β-androstan-17-one	2. The steroid sulphates were not well used by the foetal adrenal 3. This saturated steroid gave results resembling those noted with the $^5\Delta$-3β-hydroxysteroids in List 1. The authors concluded that this might mean that a Δ^5-configuration is not required for enzyme-substrate binding	
Human (1) Normal	Pregnenolone, 17α-hydroxy-pregnenolone, DHA	1 and 2. The results in normal and foetal adrenals confirm the findings of investigators 12 and 13	Calman et al. (1966)
(2) Foetal (3) Cushing's adrenals (3)	Pregnenolone sulphate 17α-hydroxypregnenolone sulphate, DHA sulphate	3. In the Cushing's adrenals studied intense 3β-hydroxysteroid dehydro-genase was noted in the zonae glomerulosa et reticularis, in addition to the usual reaction in the outer part of the zona fasciculata. The sulphates were poorly used	
(4) Adrenal adenoma		4. The adrenal adenoma closely resembled normal fascicular zone tissue in its activity	
Human foetal	DHA and DHA sulphate	Activity in neocortex with DHA only	Goldman et al. (1966)
Frog	Pregnenolone, 17α-hydroxy-pregnenolone, DHA, androstenediol	The frog adrenal cortex (Fig. 60) utilized all substrates well; no obvious zonation can be seen	M. M. Ferguson and A. H. Baillie (unpublished)
	Pregnenolone sulphate, DHA sulphate	The steroid sulphates were not used by the frog adrenal gland	
Hamster	Pregnenolone, DHA	All cortical cells (Fig. 61)	

steroid dehydrogenase is mainly localized in the outer part of the zona fasciculata; it is weakly active in the zona glomerulosa and zona reticularis; and histochemically absent from the inner half of the fascicular zone. The differences in degree described by various workers can probably be attributed to the application of different subjective standards in a field which, as yet, lacks quantitative techniques. We are unhappy, however, about the strong reactions recorded by Goldberg et al. (1963) in the zona glomerulosa of the human adrenal, because of its post-mortem collection.

The precise metabolic role of the steroid sulphates with respect to steroid hormone biosynthesis remains unknown. Several reports of direct steroid sulphate metabolism have recently been published. Of particular interest are the following conversions. (a) [³H]Pregnenolone [³⁵S]sulphate to 17α-[³H]hy-droxypregnenolone- [³⁵S]sulphate (Calvin and Lieberman, 1964) in vitro using hyperplastic adrenal homogenates. (b) Pregnenolone [³⁵S]sulphate to DHA [³⁵S]sulphate in vivo (Calvin et al., 1963). (c) [³H]Cholesterol [³⁵S]sulphate to the radioactive DHA sulphate in vivo (Roberts et al., 1964). In each instance conversion occurred without cleavage to the ester group. The limited ability of the foetal and adult adrenal cortex to metabolize DHA sulphate contrasts with the histochemical utilization of the 3β-sulphoxy derivatives of pregnenolone and 17α-hydroxypregnenolone. Evidence has recently been obtained that DHA is secreted by the adrenal cortex mainly as its sulphate ester (Baulieu, 1960; Vande Wiele *et al.*, 1963), and the limited ability of the adrenal cortex to metabolize DHA sulphate, suggested by histochemical results, may account for the secretion of this conjugate by the adrenal gland.

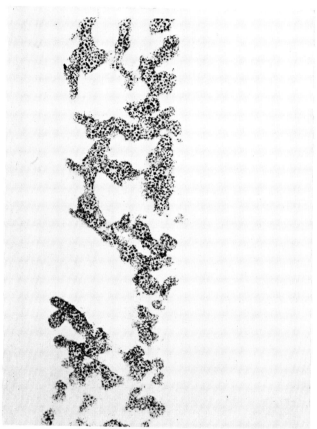

FIG. 60. (a) 3β-Hydroxysteroid dehydrogenase in all frog adrenocortical cells. Note the absence of obvious zonation. DHA was used as substrate. ×90.

All the published work to date on the histochemical localization of 3β-hydroxysteroid dehydrogenase in the adrenal relies on the use of NAD as co-factor; in this laboratory, in sections from two Cushing's adrenals, we have noted NADP-linked 3β-hydroxysteroid dehydrogenase whose distribution is the same as the NAD-linked 3β-hydroxysteroid dehydrogenase. It seems reasonable to infer from this that human adrenal 3β-hydroxysteroid dehydrogenase is not NAD-specific.

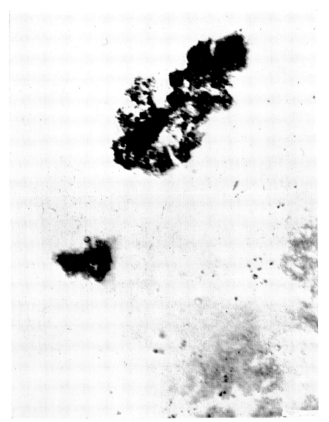

FIG. 60. Continued. (b) 3β-Hydroxysteroid dehydrogenase activity in a group of frog adrenocortical cells; a much weaker 17β-hydroxysteroid dehydrogenase reaction is present in the adjacent renal tubules. The substrate used was androstenediol. × 130.

III. 6β-Hydroxysteroid Dehydrogenase

Weak 6β-hydroxysteroid dehydrogenase activity has been recorded in the zonae fasciculata et reticularis of the rat (Baillie *et al.*, 1966), but seems to be absent from the mouse adrenal cortex (Hart *et al.*, 1966). Calman *et al.* (1966) note weak 6β-hydroxysteroid dehydrogenase activity in the foetal part of the human foetal adrenal cortex; the enzyme is virtually absent histochemically from the adult human adrenal cortex, although a trace reaction occurs in the outer part of the zona fasciculata. This trace reaction disappears in Cushing's syndrome (Calman *et al.*, 1966). 6β-Hydroxyprogesterone has been the only substrate surveyed.

IV. 11β-Hydroxysteroid Dehydrogenase

Calman *et al.* (1966) have described weak or moderate 11β-hydroxysteroid

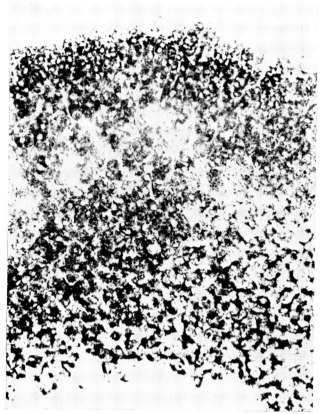

Fig. 61. 3β-Hydroxysteroid dehydrogenase activity is distributed throughout the entire hamster adrenal cortex. DHA was chosen as substrate, × 100.

dehydrogenase activity in both foetal and adult human adrenal glands. In the foetus, activity is mainly found in the foetal, as opposed to the definitive, cortex. In the adult human adrenal, 11β-hydroxysteroid dehydrogenase occurs in the outer part of the fascicular zone and in the zona reticularis. Hart *et al.* (1966) record some 11β-hydroxysteroid dehydrogenase activity in the adrenal gland of late foetal and young post-natal mice. This activity, mainly fascicular in distribution, diminishes with age. It must be clearly and unequivocally stated that in human, rat and mouse adrenal glands 11β-hydroxysteroid dehydrogenase, from a histochemical standpoint, is an extremely disappointing entity although there is biochemical evidence of its presence in various species (Haines, 1952; Rao and Heard, 1957; Hofmann and Christy, 1961; Neher *et al.*, 1962). This is not true of the hamster adrenal (Fig. 62), where intense NAD- and NADP-linked 11β-hydroxysteroid dehydrogenase activity is readily demonstrable (Ferguson and Baillie, unpublished). The peripheral zona glomerulosa shows weak 11β-hydroxysteroid dehydrogenase activity in

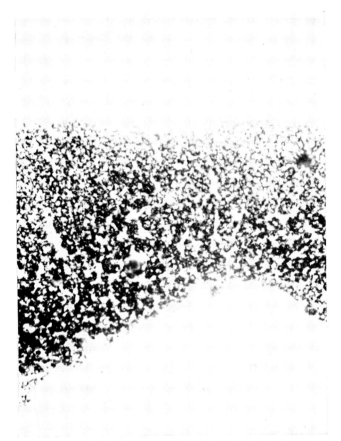

FIG. 62. 11β-Hydroxysteroid dehydrogenase activity is particularly intense in the hamster adrenal, but is restricted to the inner half of the cortex. (cf. Fig. 61). Substrate was 11β-hydroxyandrostenedione. × 100.

this species and the fasciculo-reticular zone shows a steady increase in activity as one passes centrally from the capsule.

11β-Hydroxysteroid dehydrogenase activity is present in only trace amounts histochemically in the frog adrenal gland.

V. 16α-HYDROXYSTEROID DEHYDROGENASE

This enzyme is present as *trace* activity only in the definitive human (Calman *et al.*, 1966), mouse (Hart *et al.*, 1966) and rat adrenal glands (Baillie *et al.*, 1965). Moderate activity has been noted in the foetal zone of the foetal human adrenal gland (Calman *et al.*, 1966).

VI. 16β-HYDROXYSTEROID DEHYDROGENASE

16β-Hydroxysteroids, unlike their 16α-isomers, are readily utilized histochemically by all zones of the adrenal glands of all species surveyed to date. A list of animals studied in this laboratory is given in Table 15, together with references to publications where results have previously been recorded. The

TABLE 15

Species in which histochemically demonstrable adrenal 16β- hydroxysteroid dehydrogenase is known to occur.

Human foetal adrenal	Calman *et al.* (1966)
Human adult adrenal	Calman *et al.* (1966)
Cat adrenal	Unpublished
Dog adrenal	Unpublished
Frog adrenal	Unpublished
Hamster adrenal	Unpublished
Mouse adrenal	Hart *et al.* (1966)
Rat adrenal	Baillie *et al.* (1965)

reaction is predominantly NAD-linked and its massive nature will be appreciated by reference to Figs. 63 and 64. One of the most striking features

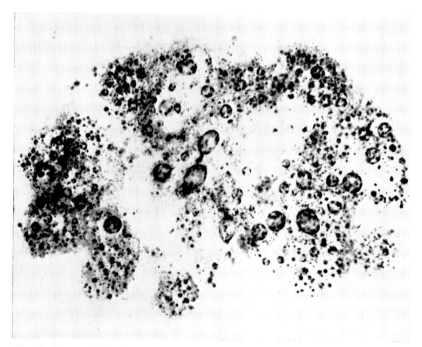

FIG. 63. Intense 16β-hydroxysteroid dehydrogenase in frog adrenocortical cells. × 270.

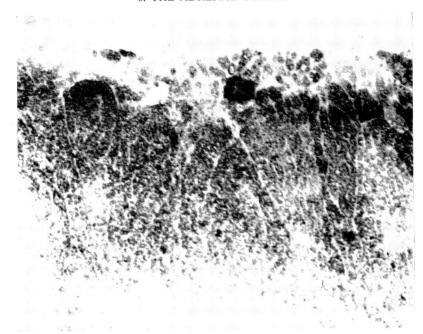

FIG. 64. Intense 16β-hydroxysteroid dehydrogenase in the zona glomerulosa of the adult human adrenal gland. × 120.

of the histochemical distribution of 16β-hydroxysteroid dehydrogenase is its intensity in the zona glomerulosa of the human adrenal gland (Fig. 64). This contrasts markedly with 3β-hydroxysteroid dehydrogenase, which is difficult to demonstrate satisfactorily in human adrenal zona glomerulosa. Moreover, in the definitive cortex of 12·4 and 17·8 cm human foetuses Calman et al. (1966) found intense 16β-hydroxysteroid dehydrogenase activity restricted to the outer part of the definitive cortex, suggesting that the most superficial cells had undergone histochemical differentiation towards definitive zona glomerulosa tissue. This point will be referred to again, when the functional significance of these data is considered.

Two points remain in connection with the distribution of this enzyme in the adrenal gland. First, in the human gland, 16β-hydroxysteroid dehydrogenase is virtually absent from the inner part of the zona fasciculata. Secondly, in the mouse the X-zone is active and in rats intensely reactive medullary rests are present. 3β, 16β-Dihydroxyandrost-5-ene 3-methyl ether is a better substrate than 16β-hydroxyoestradiol.

VII. 17β-HYDROXYSTEROID DEHYDROGENASE

Pearson and Grose (1959a, b) and Fuhrmann (1961) failed to demonstrate 17β-hydroxysteroid dehydrogenase in rodent adrenal cortex, but Levy et al.

(1959) obtained an NAD-linked colour reaction with testosterone as substrate in all zones of the rat adrenal gland. More recently Hart *et al.* (1966) noted trace activity in the zona fasciculata of mouse adrenal glands at the approach of maturity, and Calman *et al.* (1966) recorded weak 17β-hydroxysteroid dehydrogenase in human foetal and adult adrenal glands. In the foetal adrenal gland activity was confined to the foetal zone; in the adult the outer part of the zona fasciculata and the zona reticularis, were weakly reactive. Testosterone and oestradiol served as substrates and the reaction was NAD-mediated. The frog adrenal exhibits weak 17β-hydroxysteroid dehydrogenase activity.

Hydroxysteroids not used to any extent by the adrenal gland include 11α-, 12α-, 17α-, 20β-, 21- and 24-hydroxysteroids.

VIII. HYDROXYSTEROID DEHYDROGENASE DISTRIBUTION IN RELATION TO
ADRENAL ZONATION

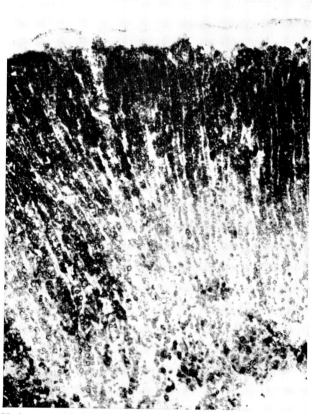

FIG. 65. 3β-Hydroxysteroid dehydrogenase is restricted to the outer part of the zona fasciculata of the human adrenal gland, with weaker activity in the zona reticularis. × 100.

In the past many workers have assumed that the visible anatomical zonation of the adrenal gland was a reflection of biochemical specialization of the different cell types in its different zones, although recently there has been a growing tendency to regard the fascicular and reticular zones as a single functional unit (Griffiths *et al.*, 1963; Griffiths and Glick, 1966). To what extent these zones are interrelated remains to be established; it is clear, however, from electron microscopic and other observations (Carr, 1962) that the cells in all three zones are morphologically distinct from one another in the human adrenal cortex, and it seems reasonable to attribute a degree of functional specialization to these different cell types.

From a phylogenetic point of view the histological and, more particularly, histochemical homogeneity of the amphibian adrenal cortex, with its uniformly distributed hydroxysteroid dehydrogenases, contrasts markedly with the human and primate adrenal cortex, where 3β-hydroxysteroid dehydrogenase is restricted mainly to the outer part of the zona fasciculata and, to a lesser

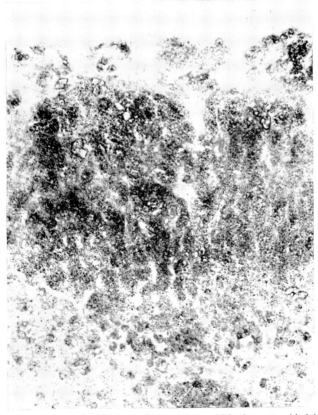

FIG. 66. In some cases of Cushing's syndrome intense 3β-hydroxysteroid dehydrogenase occurs in the zona glomerulosa. DHA was the substrate employed. × 140.

extent, to the zona reticularis (Fig. 65). In lower mammals 3β- hydroxysteroid dehydrogenase is widely distributed through all three cortical zones, and these species can perhaps be regarded as intermediate in morphology, histochemistry and function between the generalized amphibian cortex and the highly specialized primate cortex; it must be pointed out, nonetheless, that many of these lower mammals exhibit peculiar specializations of their own cortex.

Lanman (1962) expressed the view that 'the structure of the glomerular zone reflects a physiological inactivity in the foetal adrenal'. It seems clear that, although the morphological adult zones are not recognizable in the definitive part of the foetal human adrenal cortex, some degree of histochemical zonation is present at a very early stage of intra-uterine development. Thus 16β-hydroxysteroid dehydrogenase activity (Calman et al., 1966) is selectively present in the peripheral layer of cells in the foetal definitive cortex, and it seems reasonable to infer that these cells develop into the postnatal zona glomerulosa. Similarly, the inner two-thirds only of the human foetal definitive cortex exhibits 3β-hydroxysteroid dehydrogenase activity (Niemi and Baillie, 1965), and this region is presumably the precursor of the adult fascicular and reticular zones. It is not yet known whether this histochemical differentiation of the foetal definitive cortex is indicative of functional differentiation, but this would be a reasonable conclusion.

It seems to be generally agreed that the zona glomerulosa (Chester-Jones, 1957) is responsible for aldosterone biosynthesis, and there is now a considerable amount of biochemical evidence to suggest that steroids such as progesterone, 11β-hydroxyprogesterone, corticosterone and 18-hydroxycorticosterone can be converted to aldosterone by the zona glomerulosa of various animals (Ayres et al., 1956, 1957a, b, 1958; Giroud et al., 1958; Hechter, 1958; Travis and Farrell, 1958a, b; Phillips et al., 1962; Sandor and Lanthier, 1962; Sandor et al., 1963). Since normal human daily aldosterone production rates lie between 100 and 500μg according to most investigators (Chester-Jones et al., 1959; Laragh et al., 1960; Cope et al., 1961; Laumas et al., 1961; Solomon et al., 1962), with occasional maxima of from 6,000 to 10,000μg (Laragh et al., 1960) in unusual circumstances, one would not expect more than the weak 3β-hydroxysteroid dehydrogenase noted in normal human glomerulosa by most histochemists, if aldosterone production was its principal function.

Little is known of the daily aldosterone production of other mammals, and it is therefore difficult to comment on the significance of the more intense 3β-hydroxysteroid dehydrogenase activity seen histochemically in their zonae glomerulosae. It is interesting to note, however, that in the rat zona glomerulosa 3β-hydroxysteroid dehydrogenase increases histochemically if dietary sodium is restricted (Marx and Deane, 1963).

The presence of intense 16β-hydroxysteroid dehydrogenase in the human zona glomerulosa poses problems. It is difficult to relate this enzyme to any accepted schemes of steroid metabolism. Its presence in the human zona glomerulosa seems to imply that steroids other than aldosterone are metabolized in this zone, but biochemical proof of this supposition is lacking at present and it would seem wise to defer comment on the significance of this finding until such time as the biochemical role of this enzyme is better understood.

The situation with regard to the functional significance of the human fascicular and reticular zones is, unfortunately, the subject of much conflict in the literature: Chester-Jones (1957) attributes corticosteroid formation to the zona fasciculata and sex steroid formation to the zona reticularis. Symington (1960, 1962a, b) proposed a storage function for the zona fasciculata, steroid precursors being stored; Griffiths *et al.* (1963) noted that the human zona fasciculata cells contain cholesteryl ester, and suggest that such an ester may serve as a precursor of corticosteroids. The zona reticularis (Symington, 1962a) was assigned the production of 'all steroids, except aldosterone, for normal daily use'. In support of his views on the respective functions of the fascicular and reticular zones, Symington relied to some extent on the observations of Grant *et al.* (1957), who supposed that in human adrenocortical homogenates 11β-hydroxylase activity was directly proportional to the number of compact cells of reticular origin present in the homogenate. Griffiths *et al.* (1963), revising their earlier opinions, concluded that cells of the fascicular and reticular zones of the human cortex show similar steroid 11β-hydroxylating properties and accepted that the fascicular and reticular zones contributed to the daily basal secretion of cortisol and adrenal androgens.

It is against this background that the histochemical findings detailed above must be considered. Histochemically demonstrable Δ^5-3β-hydroxysteroid dehydrogenase can be regarded as strong circumstantial evidence of steroid biosynthesis, and it is quite clear that this enzymic activity is located in the outer part of the zona fasciculata, and in the zona reticularis. It is possible that this location could be determined by selective failure of steroids or co-factors to penetrate the cells of the inner part of the zona fasciculata, but poor penetration seems unlikely, in view (p, 7) of the extensive damage known to occur to cells during processing for histochemical studies. In these circumstances it seems reasonable to conclude that steroid biosynthesis occurs mainly in the outer part of the zona fasciculata and, to a slightly lesser extent, in the zona reticularis; in reaching this conclusion we must point out that the threshold of the histochemical Δ^5-3β-hydroxysteroid dehydrogenase reaction remains to be established.

Under conditions of ACTH stimulation it has been established that Δ^5-3β-hydroxysteroid dehydrogenase activity progressively appears in the inner, usually unreactive, part of the zona fasciculata. The histochemical facts imply that the bulk of steroid biosynthesis and metabolism occurs, in normal circumstances, in the outer part of the zona fasciculata, and the inner half or so of this zone in the normal human adrenal gland constitutes a relatively inactive reserve of fascicular tissue, which can be stimulated if need be. Whether this activation takes place in the outer part of the fascicular zone or at the fasciculo-reticular border, as recently suggested (Griffiths and Glick, 1966), has not yet been studied histochemically. Symington's theory that the entire zona fasciculata is principally a storage zone is clearly no longer tenable. Although Chester-Jones (1957) restricted androgen biosynthesis to the zona reticularis, the presence of 17β-hydroxysteroid dehydrogenase in the outer part of the human zona fasciculata may indicate that androgens are synthesized in both zones. This would accord with Deane's (1962) views, but the conclusion is tentative.

In lower animals it seems probable that adrenal steroid biosynthesis is active in all zones, including the mouse X-zone, and care must be taken in equating results from these species with those obtained in the primate and human adrenal cortex.

REFERENCES

Arnold, J. (1866). Ein Beitrag zu der feineren Structur und dem Chemismus der Nebennieren. *Arch. Path. Anat. Physiol.* **35**, 64–107.

Arvy, L. (1962). Présence d'une activité steroïdo-3β-ol-déshydrogénasique chez quelques Sauropsidés. *Compt. Rend.* **255**, 1803–1804.

Ayres, P. J., Gould, R. P., Simpson, S. A. and Tait, J. F. (1956). The *in vitro* demonstration of differential corticosteroid production within the ox adrenal gland. *Biochem. J.* **63**, 19p.

Ayres, P. J., Hechter, O., Saba, N., Simpson, S. A. and Tait, J. F. (1957a). Intermediates in the biosynthesis of aldosterone by capsule strippings of ox adrenal gland. *Biochem. J.* **65**, 22p.

Ayres, P. J., Garrod, O., Tait, S. A. S., Tait, J. F., Walker, G. and Pearlman, W. H. (1957b). *Ciba Found. Colloq. Endocrinol.* **11**, 309.

Ayres, P. J., Pearlman, W. H., Tait, J. F. and Tait, S. A. S. (1958). The biosynthetic preparation of (16-^{3}H) aldosterone and (16-^{3}H) corticosterone. *Biochem. J.* **70**, 230–236.

Baillie, A. H., Calman, K. C., Ferguson, M. M. and Hart, D. McK. (1966). Histochemical utilization of 3α-, 6β-, 11α-, 12α-, 16α-, 16β-, 17α-, 21- and 24-hydroxysteroids. *J. Endocrinol.* **34**, 1–12.

Baillie, A. H., Cameron, E. H. D., Griffiths, K. and Hart, D. McK. (1965). 3β-Hydroxysteroid dehydrogenase in the adrenal gland and placenta. *J. Endocrinol.* **31**, 227–233.

Baulieu, E. E. (1960). Ester-sulfates des stéroides hormonaux. Isolement de l'ester-sulfate de 5-androstène-3β-ol-17-one (déhydroépiandrosterone) dans une tumeur corticosurrénalienne. Absence du stéroide libre. *Compt. Rend.* **251**, 1421–1423.

Bloch, B., Tissenbaum, B., Rubin, B. L. and Deane, H. W. (1962). Δ^5-3β-hydroxysteroid dehydrogenase activity in human fetal adrenals. *Endocrinology* **71**, 629–632.

Calman, K. C., Baillie, A. H., Ferguson, M. M. and Hart, D. McK. (1966). Hydroxysteroid dehydrogenases in the human adrenal cortex. *J. Endocrinol.* **34**, 439–446.

Calvin, H. I. and Lieberman, S. (1964). Evidence that steroid sulfates serve as biosynthetic intermediates. II. *In vitro* conversion of pregnenolone-^{3}H sulfate-^{35}S to 17α-hydroxypregnenolone-^{3}H sulfate-^{35}S. *Biochemistry* **4**, 259–264.

Calvin, H. I., Vande Wiele, R. L. and Lieberman, S. (1963). Evidence that steroid sulfates serve as biosynthetic intermediates: *In vivo* conversion of pregnenolone-sulfate-^{35}S to dehydroisoandrosterone-sulfate-^{35}S. *Biochemistry* 2, 648–653.

Carr, I. A. (1962). The electron microscopy of the adrenal cortex. In: *The human adrenal cortex* (Ed. Currie, Symington and Grant), pp. 21–25 (Livingstone, Edinburgh).

Cavallero, C. and Chiappino, G. (1961). Istologia ed istochimica della corteccia surrenale negli ipercorticalismi. *IX Congresso Nationale. Simposia su la m. di Cushing, Soc. Ital. Endocrinol.* p. 5 (Arti Graphiche Pacini Mariotti, Pisa).

Cavallero, C. and Chiappino, G. (1962). Histochemistry of steroid-3β-ol dehydro-genase in the human adrenal cortex. *Experientia* 18, 119–120.

Cavallero, M. C., Magrini, U., Dellepiane, M. and Cizely, T. (1965). Étude histo-chimique du cortex surrénalien et du testicule chez le foetus humain. *Ann. Endocrinol. (Paris)* 26, 409–418.

Chester-Jones, I. (1957). *The adrenal cortex.* (Cambridge University Press).

Chester-Jones, I., Lloyd-Jones, R., Riondel, A., Tait, J. F., Tait, S. A. S., Bulbrook, R. D. and Greenwood, F. C. (1959). Aldosterone secretion and metabolism in normal men and women and in pregnancy. *Acta Endocrinol.* 30, 321–342.

Cope, C. L., Nicolis, G. and Fraser, B. (1961). Measurement of aldosterone secretion rate in man by the use of a metabolite. *Clin. Sci.* 21, 367–380.

Dawson, I. M. P., Pryse-Davies, J. and Snape, I. M. (1961a). The histochemical demonstration of steroid 3β-ol dehydrogenase and diphosphopyridine nucleo-tide diaphorase in the adrenal cortex. *Biochem. J.* 78, 16p.

Dawson, I. M. P., Pryse-Davies, J. and Snape, I. M. (1961b). The distribution of six enzyme systems and of lipid in the human and rat adrenal cortex before and after administration of steroid and ACTH, with comments on the distribution in human foetuses and in some natural disease conditions. *J. Path. Bact.* 81, 181–195

Deane, H. W. (1962). In: *Handb. Exp. Pharmacol., Erg. W.* Bdn, XIV/1 (Springer, Berlin).

Freses, A. T., Diaz, J. and Falen, J. (1965). Efecto de ACTH, dexametasona y progesterona sobre la actividad de 3β-ol-esteroide deshidrogenaxe de la suprarrenal de rata albina. Estudio histoquimico. *Rev. Iber. Endocrinol.* 12, 5–14.

Fuhrmann, K. (1961). Uber den histochemischen Nachweis der 3β-ol-Steroid-dehydrogenase-aktivitat in Geweben endokriner Organe. *Zentr. Gynaekol.* 15, 565–572.

Fuhrmann, K. (1963). Histochemische Untersuchungen uber Hydroxysteroid Dehydrogenase-Aktivitat in Nebennieren und Eierstocken von Ratten und Kaninchen *Arch Gynaekol* 197, 583–600

Giroud, C. J. P., Stachenko, J. and Piletta, P. (1958). In: *Aldosterone* (Ed. A. F. Muller and C. M. O'Connor), p. 56. (Little, Brown, Boston, Mass.).

Goldberg, B., Jones, G. E. and Turner, D. A. (1963). Steroid 3β-ol dehydrogenase activity in human endocrine tissues. *Am. J. Obstet. Gynecol.* 86, 349–359.

Goldman, A. S., Yakovac, W. C. and Bongiovanni, A. M. (1965). Persistent effects of a synthetic androstene derivative on activities of 3β-hydroxysteroid dehydro-genase and glucose-6-phosphate dehydrogenase in rats. *Endocrinol.* 77, 1105–1118.

Goldman, A. S., Yakovac, W. C. and Bongiovanni, A. M. (1966). Development of activity of 3β-hydroxysteroid dehydrogenase in human fetal tissues and in two anencephalic newborns. *J. Clin. Endocrinol. Metab.* 26, 14–22.

Goldman, A. S., Bongiovanni, A. M. Yakovac W. C. and Prader, A. (1964). Study of Δ^5, 3β-HSD in normal, hyperplastic and neoplastic adrenal cortical tissue. *J. Clin. Endocrinol. Metab.* **24**, 894–909.

Gottschau, M. (1883). Structur und embryonale Entwickelung der Nebennieren bei Saugethieren. *Arch. Anat. Entwicklngsgesch. Leipz.* 412–418.

Grant, J. K., Symington, T. and Duguid, W. P. (1957). Effect of adrenocorticotropic therapy on the *in vitro* 11β-hydroxylation of deoxycorticosterone by human adrenal homogenates. *J. Clin. Endocrinol. Metab.* **17**, 933.

Griffiths, K. and Glick, D. (1966). Determination of 11β-hydroxylase activity in microgram samples of tissue, its quantitative histological distribution in the rat adrenal influence of ACTH. *J. Endocrinol.* (in press).

Griffiths, K., Grant, J. K. and Symington, T. (1963). A biochemical investigation of the functional zonation of the adrenal cortex in man. *J. Clin. Endocrinol. Metab.* **23**, 776–785.

Haines, W. J. (1952). Studies on the biosynthesis of adrenal cortex hormones. *Recent Progr. Hormone Res.* **7**, 255–305.

Hart, D. McK., Baillie, A. H., Calman, K. C. and Ferguson, M. M. (1966). Hydroxysteroid dehydrogenase development in mouse adrenal and gonads. *J. Anat. London* **100** (in press).

Hechter, O. (1958). In: *Cholesterol* (Ed. R. P. Cook), p. 309. (Academic Press, New York).

Hofmann, F. G. and Christy, N. P. (1961). Studies *in vitro* of steroid hormone biosynthesis. *Biochim. Biophys. Acta.* **54**, 354–356.

Lanman, J. T. (1962). An interpretation of human foetal adrenal structure and function. In: *The human adrenal cortex* (Ed. Currie, Symington and Grant) Livingstone, Edinburgh pp. 547–558.

Laragh, J. H., Ulick, S., Januszewicz, V., Deming, Q. B., Kelly, W. G. and Lieberman, S. (1960). Aldosterone secretion and primary and malignant hypertension. *J. Clin. Invest.* **39**, 1091–1106.

Laumas, K. R., Tait, J. F. and Tait, S. A. S. (1961). The validity of the calculation of secretion rates from the specific activity of a urinary metabolite. *Acta Endocrinol.* **36**, 265–280.

Levy, H., Deane, H. W. and Rubin, B. L. (1959). Visualization of steroid-3β-ol-dehydrogenase activity in tissues of intact and hypophysectomized rats. *Endocrinology* **65**, 932–943.

Marx, A. H. and Deane, H. W. (1963). Histophysiologic changes in the kidney and adrenal cortex in rats on a low-sodium diet. *Endocrinology* **73**, 317–328.

Marx, A. J., Deane, H. W., Mowles, T. F. and Sheppard, H. (1963). Chronic administration of angiotensin in rats: changes in blood pressure, renal and adrenal histophysiology and aldosterone production. *Endocrinology* **73**, 329–337.

Narbaitz, R. and Kolodny, L. (1964). Δ^5-3β-Hydroxysteroid dehydrogenase in differentiating chick gonads. *Z. Zellfarsch* **63**, 612–617.

Neher, R., Roversi, G. D., Polvani, F. and Bompiani, A. (1962). *Excerpta Med. Intern. Congr. Ser.* **51**, 237.

Niemi, M. and Baillie, A. H. (1965). 3β-Hydroxysteroid dehydrogenase activity in the human foetal adrenal cortex. *Acta Endocrinol.* **48**, 423–428.

Pearson, B. and Grose, F. (1959a). Histochemical study of some DPNH and DPN dependent dehydrogenases. *Federation Proc.* **18**, 499.

Pearson, B. and Grose, F. (1959b). Histochemical demonstration of 17β-hydroxy-steroid dehydrogenase by use of tetrazolium salt. *Proc. Soc. Exptl. Biol. Med.* **100**, 636–638.

Pearson, B., Wolf, P., Grose, F. and Andrews, M. (1964). The histochemistry of 3β-hydroxysteroid dehydrogenase. I. With special reference to adrenal glands, as affected by ACTH, cold, traumal tumor. *Am. J. Clin. Path.* **41**, 256–265.

Phillips, J. G., Chester-Jones, I. and Bellamy, D. (1962). Biosynthesis of adrenocortical hormones by adrenal glands of lizards and snakes. *J. Endocrinol.* **25**, 233–237.

Price, D., Ortiz, E. and Deane, H. W. (1964). The presence of Δ⁵-3β-hydroxysteroid dehydrogenase in fetal guinea pig testes and adrenal glands. *Am. Zool.* **4**, No. 4.

Rao, B. H. and Heard, R. D. H. (1957). Biogenesis of the corticosteroids. II. Conversion of C¹⁴-progesterone in cell-free hog adrenal preparations. *Arch. Biochem. Biophys.* **66**, 504–505.

Roberts, K. D., Bandi, L., Calvin, H. I., Drucker, W. D. and Lieberman, S. (1964). Evidence that cholesterol sulfate is a precursor of steroid hormones. *J. Am. Chem. Soc.* **86**, 958–959.

Rubin, B. L., Deane, H. W. and Hamilton, J. A. (1963). Biochemical and histo-chemical studies on Δ⁵-3β-hydroxysteroid dehydrogenase activity in the adrenal glands and ovaries of diverse mammals. *Endocrinology* **73**, 748–763.

Sandor, T. and Lanthier, A. (1962). The metabolism of aldosterone. II. Studies *in vitro* and *in vivo* in man. *Acta Endocrinol.* **39**, 87–102.

Sandor, T., Lanthier, A. and Lamoureux, J. (1963). The *in vitro* biosynthesis of radioactive steroids by the adrenals of the domestic duck and pond turtle. *Federation Proc.* **22**, 270.

Solomon, S., Watanabe, M., Dominguez, O. V., Gray, M. J., Meeker, C. I. and Simms, E. A. H. (1962). *Excerpta Med. Intern. Congr. Ser.* **51**, 267.

Symington, T. (1960). The morphology of the adrenal cortex. *Biochem. Soc. Symposia* **18**, 40–49.

Symington, T. (1962a). The morphology and zoning of the human adrenal cortex. In: *The human adrenal cortex* (Ed. Currie, Symington and Grant) (Livingstone, Edinburgh).

Symington, T. (1962b). Morphology and secretory cytology of the human adrenal cortex. *Brit. Med. Bull.* **18**, 117–121.

Travis, R. H. and Farrell, G. L. (1958a). *In vitro* biosynthesis of isotopic aldosterone: comparison of precursors. *Endocrinology* **63**, 882–886.

Travis, R. H. and Farrell, G. L. (1958b). Precursors of Aldosterone; *In vitro* studies. *Federation Proc.* **17**, 324.

Vande Wiele, R. L., MacDonald, P. C., Bolte, E. and Lieberman, S. (1963). Precursors of the urinary 11-desoxy-17-ketosteroids: estimation of the secretory rate of dehydroisoandrosterone. *J. Clin. Endocrinol.* **22**, 1207–1221.

Wattenberg, L. W. (1958). Microscopic histochemical demonstration of steroid-3β-ol-dehydrogenase in tissue sections. *J. Histochem. Cytochem.* **6**, 225–232.

CHAPTER 7

The Renal System

I. The Pronephros

Some lower chordates retain a functioning pronephros throughout adult life; so far as we can determine, the distribution of hydroxysteroid dehydrogenases has not been studied in such primitive forms. The mammalian pronephros has a brief existence, and consists, at the height of its development, of a number, described variously as from 7 to 14, of tubules in the cervical area of the embryo. The human pronephros possesses no histochemically demonstrable hydroxysteroid dehydrogenases (Baillie *et al.*, 1966a).

II. The Mesonephros

The mesonephros is the functional kidney in many fish and amphibia. A

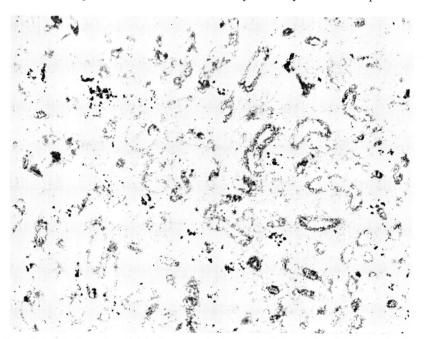

Fig. 67. 17β-Hydroxysteroid dehydrogenase in the renal tubules of the plaice, after incubation with oestradiol. × 100.

histochemically active 17β-hydroxysteroid dehydrogenase can be demonstrated in most fish mesonephroi (Table 17(a), Fig. 67) and in amphibian mesonephroi (Fig. 68) (Baillie *et al.*, 1966a). The mesonephric 17β-hydroxy-

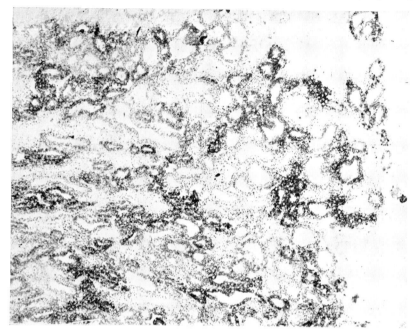

FIG. 68. 17β-Hydroxysteroid dehydrogenase in the mesonephros of the common frog, after incubation with testosterone. × 180.

steroid dehydrogenase exhibits a marked substrate preference for testosterone but oestradiol and 17β-hydroxy-5α-androstan are also utilized (Table 16).

3α-Hydroxysteroid dehydrogenase occurs in histochemically demonstrable amounts in one or two fish mesonephroi (Table 17(a)) but seems to be absent

TABLE 16

Substrate specificity of plaice kidney 17β-hydroxysteroid dehydrogenase. The reaction intensity was judged visually and is denoted by a simple +, − system.

Testosterone	+ +
Oestradiol	+
17β-Hydroxy-5α-androstan-3-one	+
17β-Hydroxy-5β-androstan-3-one	−
Testosterone propionate	−
Testosterone phenylpropionate	−
Testosterone isocaproate	trace
Testosterone decanoate	−
Testosterone sulphate	−

E

TABLE 17(a)

Vertebrate kidney: phylogenetic study

Animal	Type of kidney	Hydroxysteroid dehydrogenase investigated							
		3α	Δ⁵-3β	6β	11β	16α	16β	17β	20β
Dogfish—*Scyliorhinus canicula*	Mesonephros	−	−	−	−	−	−	+	−
Skate—*Raja batis*	Mesonephros	+	−	−	−	−	−	−	−
Sea Scorpion—*Cottus bubalis*	Mesonephros	trace	−	−	−	−	−	+	−
Cod—*Gadus morhua*	Mesonephros	trace	−	−	−	−	−	+	−
Whiting—*Gadus merlangus*	Mesonephros	−	−	−	−	−	−	+	−
Plaice—*Platessa platessa*	Mesonephros	−	−	−	−	−	+	+	−
Frog—*Rana temporaria*	Mesonephros	−	−	−	−	−	trace	+¹	−
Tortoise—*Testudo graeca*	Metanephros	+¹	−	−	−	+¹	+¹	+¹	−
Chicken—*Gallus domesticus*	Metanephros	+¹	−	−	+³	−	trace	+¹	−
Rat—*Rattus rattus*	Metanephros	+²	trace	−	+³	−	trace	+¹	−
Mouse—*Mus Muris*	Metanephros	+²	trace	trace	+³	−	trace	+¹	−
Cat—*Felis catus*	Metanephros	+²	trace	trace	+³	trace	+¹	+¹	−
Dog—*Canis familiaris*	Metanephros	+²	trace	trace	+³	+¹	+¹	+¹	−
Guinea-pig—*Cavia porcellus*	Metanephros	+²	trace	trace	+³	−	+¹	+¹	−
Cow—*Bos taurus*	Metanephros	−	trace	trace	+³	−	trace	+¹	−
Pig—*Sus scrofa*	Metanephros	trace	−	−	+³	−	−	+¹	−
Hamster—*Mesocricetus auratus*	Metanephros	+²	trace	trace	+³	−	+¹	+¹	−
Monkey—*Rhesus macacus*	Metanephros	trace	−	−	+³	trace	trace	trace¹	−

[1] Hydroxysteroid dehydrogenase activity noted in entire nephron.

[2] Hydroxysteroid dehydrogenase activity located mainly in the proximal and distal convoluted tubules.

[3] Hydroxysteroid dehydrogenase activity confined to the collecting tubules.

TABLE 17(b)

Human kidney: ontogenetic study

	3α-	Δ⁵-3β-	6β-	11β-	16α-	16β-	17β-	20β-
				Hydroxysteroid dehydrogenase investigated				
Pronephros, 14 mm foetus	—	—	—	—	—	—	—	—
Mesonephros, 14 mm foetus 45 mm 75 mm	—	trace	—	—	—	+[1]	+[1]	—
Metanephros, 110 mm 190 mm foetuses	trace	—	—	trace	—	—	—	—
Metanephros, adult	+ poor[2]	trace[1]	—	+[3]	—	+ poor[1]	+ poor[1]	trace

[1] Hydroxysteroid dehydrogenase activity noted in the entire nephron.
[2] Hydroxysteroid dehydrogenase activity mainly located in the proximal and distal convoluted tubules.
[3] Hydroxysteroid dehydrogenase activity confined to the collecting tubules.

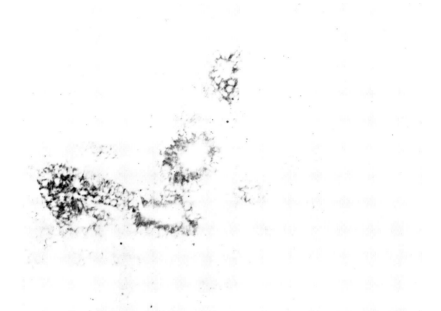

FIG. 69. 17β-Hydroxysteroid dehydrogenase in human mesonephric tubules from a 14 mm embryo. Testosterone was used as substrate. × 200.

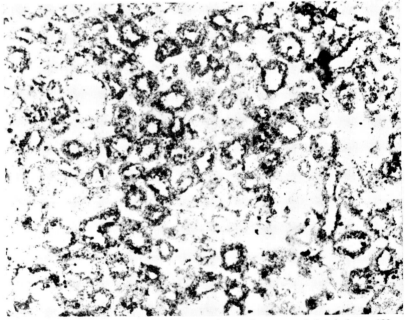

FIG. 70. 16β-Hydroxysteroid dehydrogenase in tortoise metanephric tubules. × 180.

from the amphibian mesonephros, if the frog is at all representative. It therefore cannot be considered a constant feature of the mesonephros. 16β-Hydroxysteroid dehydrogenase (Table 17(a)) is present in one fish and one amphibian mesonephros. It is not a particularly active enzyme, histochemically. The functional significance of these enzymes will be considered when their distribution in the metanephros has been reviewed.

The mesonephros of a 14 mm human embryo (Baillie *et al.*, 1966a) possessed extremely active 16β- and 17β-hydroxysteroid dehydrogenases in its tubules (Fig. 69, Table 17(b)) together with trace 3β-hydroxysteroid dehydrogenase. It is therefore clear that the transient mammalian mesonephros is histochemically similar to the mesonephroi of other lower vertebrates.

The functional status of the mesonephros in mammals varies enormously: the rat mesonephros (Torrey, 1961) is rudimentary, whereas the pig mesone-

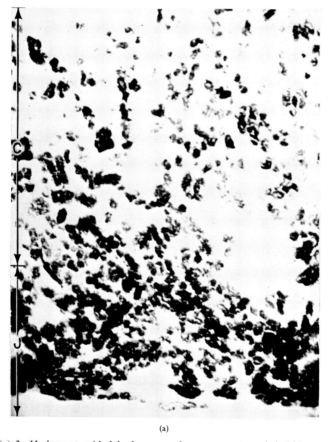

(a)

Fig. 71. (a) 3α-Hydroxysteroid dehydrogenase in mouse metanephric kidney convoluted tubules. The tubules arising from juxta-medullary glomeruli (J) stain more intensely than the rest of the cortical nephrons (C). × 70.

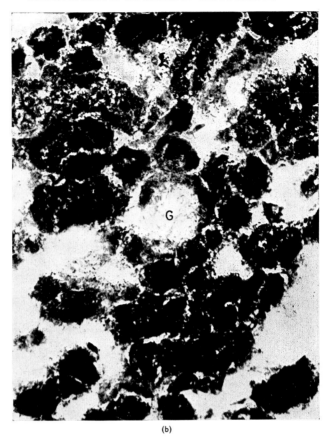

(b)

Fig. 71. Continued. (b) An unreactive glomerulus (G) surrounded by proximal and distal
convoluted tubules showing intense 3α-hydroxysteroid dehydrogenase activity. × 350.

phros exhibits both glomerular and tubular function. Histologically the
embryonic human mesonephros falls between these two extremes, but the
histochemical findings point to the possibility that the human mesonephros,
from the point of steroid excretion at least, is functional.

III. METANEPHROS

The earliest (from the phylogenetic point of view) metanephric kidney
examined histochemically is the reptilian kidney (Table 17(a)). Already 3α-,
16α-, 16β- and 17β-hydroxysteroid dehydrogenases are demonstrable in the
renal tubules (Fig. 70).

This pattern of hydroxysteroid dehydrogenase activity is evident in all the
metanephric kidneys studied in this laboratory (Baillie *et al.*, 1966a, b;

Baillie, 1966; Ferguson, 1966) but with progressive phylogenetic evolution the following changes occur.

(1) *The range of hydroxysteroid dehydrogenase activity exhibited by the nephron increases.* Weak 3β- and 6β-hydroxysteroid dehydrogenases become demonstrable; a strong 11β-hydroxysteroid dehydrogenase appears in avian metanephroi.

(2) *Increasing functional zonation of the nephron becomes apparent.* For example, 3α-hydroxysteroid dehydrogenase, which in the reptilian metanephric kidney exhibited a general distribution throughout the nephron, becomes more or less confined to the proximal and distal convoluted tubules (Fig. 71). Goldman *et al.* (1965) noted 3α-hydroxysteroid dehydrogenase activity in rat kidneys but make no reference to its location. An even more striking example of this functional organization of the nephron is the change observed in 11β-hydroxysteroid dehydrogenase distribution. When this enzyme first appears in the avian kidney it can be detected histochemically in all parts (Fig. 72) of the nephron. In all mammalian kidneys, including primate and

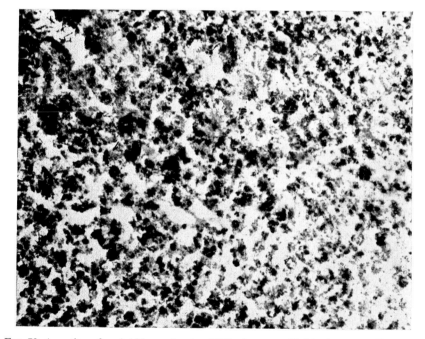

FIG. 72. A section of cock kidney, showing 11β-hydroxysteroid dehydrogenase distributed throughout the nephron. × 80.

human kidneys, the 11β-hydroxysteroid dehydrogenase becomes restricted to the collecting tubules in the cortex (Fig. 73). Moreover, in collecting tubules exhibiting 11β-hydroxysteroid dehydrogenase activity two cell types can be recognized. By far the commonest is a cell possessing strong 11β-hydroxysteroid dehydrogenase activity (Fig. 74), but interspersed with these reactive

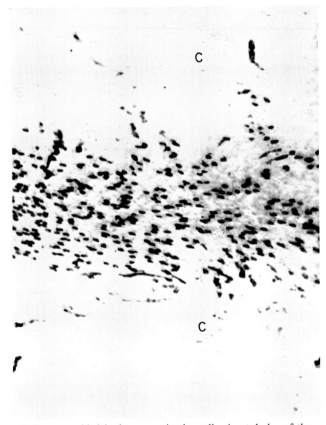

FIG. 73. 11β-Hydroxysteroid dehydrogenase in the collecting tubules of the mouse metanephros. A few are seen in the cortex (C); the majority are cut in transverse section as they leave the cortex. × 80.

cells in the wall of the collecting tubule are large cells which show no evidence of 11β-hydroxysteroid dehydrogenase activity. The relationship of these cell types to one another is unclear.

(3) *There is some evidence of functional specialization between the nephrons themselves.* This is most marked in the mouse where 3α-hydroxysteroid dehydrogenase is extremely strong in nephrons arising from the juxtamedullary glomeruli, and, by contrast, nephrons arising elsewhere in the cortex exhibit a much weaker 3α-hydroxysteroid dehydrogenase.

Most of the renal hydroxysteroid dehydrogenases utilize either NAD or NADP histochemically; hydroxysteroid dehydrogenases giving a weak

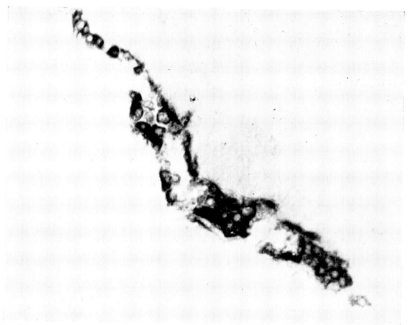

FIG. 74. A high-power view of a human collecting tubule, showing intense 11β-hydroxy-steroid dehydrogenase activity in some cells of the tubule wall while others are unreactive.
× 400.

reaction, such as 3β-hydroxysteroid dehydrogenase, are NAD-linked, and it is not clear whether this is a true reflection of the enzyme's pyridine nucleotide requirements or whether this apparent specificity is imposed by the sensitivity threshold of the reaction.

Human foetal metanephric kidneys exhibit histochemically demonstrable 11β-hydroxysteroid dehydrogenase activity. In the foetal mouse, the meta-nephric kidney 17β-hydroxysteroid dehydrogenase is the first to appear histo-chemically and becomes demonstrable during foetal life. 11β-Hydroxysteroid dehydrogenase is the last to appear and only becomes well developed some time after birth in the mouse. It may also be said of the mammalian meta-nephric kidney that ontogeny repeats phylogeny, in histochemical terms at least.

IV. BIOCHEMICAL AND FUNCTIONAL CONSIDERATIONS

3α-Hydroxysteroid dehydrogenases from bacterial or mammalian sources appear to be specific for the 3α-hydroxyl group of 5α- and 5β-steroids. 3α-Hydroxysteroid dehydrogenase has been isolated from mouse, rat, guinea-pig, rabbit and dog livers and kidneys (Hurlock and Talalay, 1958; Koide, 1963; Baron et al., 1963; Villee and Loring, 1963; Aoshima et al., 1964), and with its dual nucleotide specificity both biochemically (Hurlock and Talalay, 1958; Baron et al., 1963) and histochemically (Baillie et al., 1966a, b) has been ascribed a transhydrogenase function.

A wide variety of 3α-hydroxysteroids occur naturally in human and other urine, including aetiocholanolone, androsterone, 11β-hydroxyaetiocholanolone, 11β-hydroxyandrosterone, 11-oxoaetiocholanolone, 11-oxoandrosterone and various corresponding progesterone and other derivatives. Many of these urinary steroids (Birchall et al., 1963) represent the excretion products of Δ⁴-3-keto steroids, and the probable mechanism of excretion is summarized

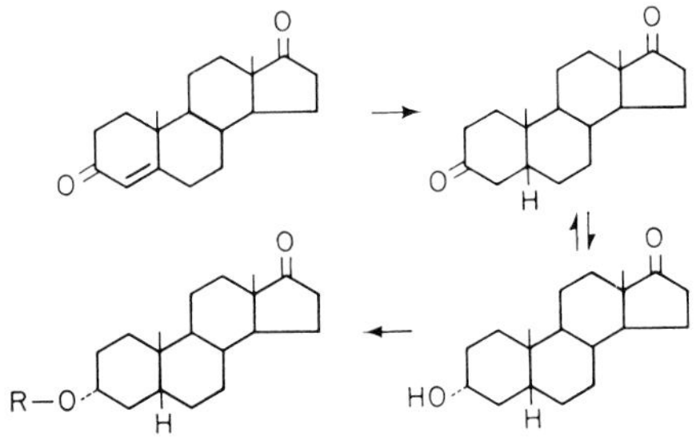

FIG. 75. A possible role for 3α-hydroxysteroid dehydrogenase in the excretion of Δ⁴-3-keto steroids.

in Fig. 75. The 3α-hydroxysteroids may be excreted in a free or esterified state, and the histochemical findings suggest that excretion of Δ⁴-3-keto steroids by the route proposed in Fig. 75 occurs throughout the nephron in lower vertebrates and is more or less selectively accomplished in the proximal and distal convoluted tubules of mammalian metanephric kidneys. The particular strength of the 3α-hydroxysteroid dehydrogenase reaction in the convoluted tubules of juxta-medullary glomeruli raises the possibility that inner and outer cortical nephrons behave rather differently with respect to steroid excretion, but further work is needed to elucidate this point.

Cathro et al. (1963) have shown that in the human infant 3α-hydroxysteroids such as aetiocholanolone or androsterone are only excreted in small amounts in the urine and this accords with the weak 3α-hydroxysteroid dehydrogenase noted histochemically in human foetal kidneys.

Wattenberg (1958) failed to observe Δ⁵-3β-hydroxysteroid dehydrogenase histochemically in the rabbit kidney, and the reaction observed in the various kidneys examined in this laboratory using Δ⁵-3β-hydroxysteroids as substrates (Table 16) is minimal or absent. Since this enzyme is more usually associated with steroidogenesis, its poor development in the kidney is hardly surprising. 3β-Hydroxysteroid dehydrogenase has, however, been recorded biochemically in renal tissue, and 3β-hydroxy-5β-steroids are utilized histochemically (p. 12).

A variety of 6β-hydroxy- and 6-ketosteroids occur in human urine in small amounts (Cathro et al., 1965) and 6β-hydroxysteroid dehydrogenase is not a convincing histochemical entity in the kidney; the substrate used in our various investigations was 6β-hydroxyprogesterone and it may be that a more suitable histochemical substrate exists.

The selective localization of the massive NAD- and NADP-linked 11β-hydroxysteroid dehydrogenase in the collecting tubules of the mammalian and primate kidneys studied is the most striking feature of renal hydroxysteroid dehydrogenase histochemistry. Biochemical precedents for this renal 11β-hydroxysteroid dehydrogenase exist (Mahesh and Ulrich, 1959; Mahesh, 1960; Koerner and Hellman, 1964), but these studies to date have tended to concentrate on the oxidation of cortisol to cortisone and have ignored to a greater or lesser extent the ability of the enzyme to deal with other physiologically active steroids such as the 11β-hydroxyandrogens. The histochemical data would suggest that the ability to metabolize, and possibly excrete, 11β-hydroxysteroids is first well developed in the avian renal tubule and becomes progressively restricted to the collecting tubules of the mammalian kidney. This point emphasizes the growing belief in recent years that the collecting tubules are more than inert tubes. Moreover (Chapter 9, p. 135), the observed 11β-hydroxysteroid dehydrogenase activity in the collecting tubules may be relevant to corticosteroid control of sodium and potassium excretion.

Mahesh and Ulrich (1959) record that cortisol–cortisone oxidation in rat renal homogenates occurs mainly in fractions containing microsomes and nuclear particles, and does not take place in the mitochondrial fraction or in the supernatant. Light microscope resolution with the existing techniques is such that intracellular localization is not possible, and we cannot offer comment on the localization of Mahesh and Ulrich (1959).

16α-Hydroxysteroid dehydrogenase occurs in female rat kidneys biochemically (Ryan et al., 1963). Histochemically there is considerable species variation in the strength of 16α-hydroxysteroid dehydrogenase activity in the kidneys; its physiological role is unclear. Biochemical knowledge of the role of 16β-hydroxysteroid dehydrogenase in the kidney is equally unsatisfactory, and again in the histochemical findings point to substantial species variations in the distribution of this enzyme.

17β-Hydroxysteroid dehydrogenase, known biochemically to exist in the kidney (Endahl et al., 1960; Velle and Erichsen, 1960; Endahl and Kochakian, 1962; Aoshima and Kochakian, 1963), can now be assigned to the convoluted tubules, and, to a lesser extent, to the loops of Henle. On the basis of these histochemical observations it seems reasonable to assume that the interconversion of oestradiol and oestrone, androstenedione and testosterone, androstenediol and DHA, and similar pairs of steroids, occurs throughout the nephron, although predominantly in the convoluted tubules. Such interconversions are relevant to the excretion of 17-keto steroids and 17-hydroxysteroids, which appears, therefore, to be carried out by the entire nephron and principally the convoluted tubules. There is some evidence (Dorfman and Ungar, 1965) that there are multiple enzymes with varying pyridine nucleotide requirements and differing locations in the cellular fractions of the guinea-pig kidney.

20β, 21- and 24-Hydroxysteroid dehydrogenases are not histochemically demonstrable in the kidneys surveyed in this laboratory.

REFERENCES

Aoshima, Y. and Kochakian, C. D. (1963). Activity, intracellular distribution and some properties of 17β-hydroxy-C-19-steroid dehydrogenases in liver and kidney. *Endocrinology* **72**, 106–114.

Aoshima, Y., Kochakian, C. D. and Jadrijevic, (1964). TPN and DPN-specific 3β-hydroxy and Δ⁵-3β-hydroxysteroid dehydrogenases of liver and kidney. *Endocrinology* **74**, 521–531.

Baillie, A. H. (1966). Histochemical evidence suggesting steroid excretion in the nephron. *J. Endocrinol.* **34**, XVIII.

Baillie, A. H., Ferguson, M. M. and Hart, D. McK. (1966a). Ontogenetic distribution of hydroxysteroid dehydrogenases in human pro-, meso- and metanephric kidneys; phylogenetic distribution of hydroxysteroid dehydrogenases in the vertebrate kidney. *J. Endocrinol* (in press).

Baillie, A. H., Calman, K. C., Ferguson, M. M. and Hart, D. McK. (1966b). Histochemical distribution of hydroxysteroid dehydrogenases in kidney and liver. *Histochemie* **5**, 384–395.

Baron, D. N., Gore, M. B. R., Pietruszko, R. and Williams, D. C. (1963). Purification and properties of the 3α-hydroxysteroid-dependent nicotinamide-adenine dinucleotide transhydrogenase of rat liver. *Biochem. J.* **88**, 19–25.

Birchall, K., Cathro, D. M., Forsyth, C. C. and Mitchell, F. L. (1963). A method for the separation and estimation of neutral steroids in the urine of newborn infants. *J. Endocrinol.* **27**, 31–51.

Cathro, D. M., Birchall, K., Mitchell, F. L. and Forsyth, C. C. (1963). The excretion of neutral steroids in the urine of newborn infants. *J. Endocrinol.* **27**, 53–75.

Dorfman, R. I. and Ungar, F. (1965). *Metabolism of steroid hormones* (Academic Press, New York).

Endahl, G. L. and Kochakian, C. D. (1962). Partial purification and further characterization of the triphosphopyridine nucleotide specific C¹⁹-17β-hydroxysteroid dehydrogenase of guinea-pig liver. *Biochim. Biophys. Acta.* **62**, 245–250.

Endahl, G. L., Kochakian, C. D. and Hamm, D. (1960). Separation of a TPN-specific from a DPN-specific 17β-hydroxy (testosterone) dehydrogenase of guinea-pig liver. *J. Biol. Chem.* **235**, 2792–2796.

Ferguson, M. M. (1966). *J. Anat.* (in press).

Goldman, A. S., Yakovac, W. C. and Bongiovanni, A. M. (1965). Persistent effects of a synthetic androstene derivative on activities of 3β-hydroxysteroid dehydrogenase and glucose-6-phosphate dehydrogenase in rats. *Endocrinology* **77**, 1105–1118.

Hurlock, B. and Talalay, P. (1958). 3α-Hydroxysteroids as co-enzymes of hydrogen transfer between di- and tri-phosphopyridine nucleotides. *J. Biol. Chem.* **233**, 886–897.

Koerner, D. R. and Hellman, L. (1964). Effect of thyroxine administration on the 11β-hydroxysteroid dehydrogenase in rat liver and kidney. *Endocrinology* **75**, 592–601.

Koide, S. S. (1963). Purification of 3α-hydroxysteroid dehydrogenase obtained from the soluble fraction of rat liver. *Arch. Biochem.* **101**, 278–285.

Mahesh, V. B. (1960). *In vitro* metabolism of steroids in the rat kidney. *Federation Proc.* **29**, 174.

Mahesh, V. B. and Ulrich, F. (1959). Distribution of enzyme systems responsible for steroid metabolism in different tissues and subcellular fractions. *Nature* **184**, 1147–1148.

Ryan, K. J. R., Meigs, A., Petro, Z. and Morrison, G. (1963). Estrogen induced 16-hydroxysteroid dehydrogenase activity in rat kidney. *Science* **142**, 243.

Torrey, W. (1961). *Morphogenesis of the vertebrates* pp. 362–406 (Wiley, New York).

Velle, W. and Erichsen, S. (1960). Studies on oestrogens in cattle. *Acta Endocrinol.* **33**, 277–286.

Villee, C. A. and Loring, J. M. (1963). 20α-Hydroxysteroid dehydrogenase and 3α-hydroxysteroid dehydrogenase in human foetal liver. *Endocrinology* **72**, 824–828.

Wattenberg, L. W. (1958). Microscopic histochemical demonstration of steroid-3β-ol dehydrogenase in tissue sections. *J. Histochem. Cytochem.* **6**, 225–232.

CHAPTER 8

The Alimentary Tract

I. SALIVARY GLANDS

With the exception of striated ducts, which are considered possibly to influence the salivary water and calcium content (Maximow and Bloom, 1942), the ducts from the mucous and serous cells of salivary glands have hitherto been thought to function as passive conduits for saliva into the oral cavity.

In rat, mouse and rabbit parotid and submandibular salivary glands the striated, intralobular and interlobular ducts exhibit 11β-hydroxysteroid dehydrogenase only, utilizing cortisol and 11β-hydroxy androstenedione as substrates (M. M. Ferguson, unpublished). The remaining acinar tissue shows no significant reaction (Fig. 76).

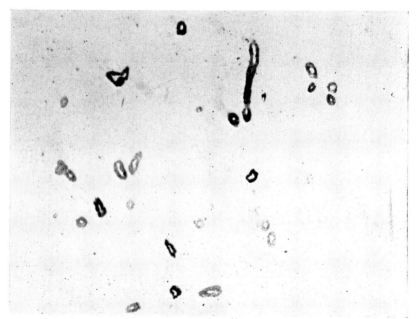

FIG. 76. 11β-Hydroxysteroid dehydrogenase activity in the ducts of the rat submandibular salivary glands, with cortisol as substrate. $\times$ 60.

The salivary concentrations of sodium and potassium in man vary in a daily rhythm, the Na^+ : K^+ ratio being highest just prior to wakening and lowest about mid-day (Grad, 1951: de Traverse and Coquelet, 1952). The relationship noted between plasma ACTH and the salivary $Na^+ : K^+$ ratio suggests that corticosteroids other than aldosterone influence this ratio (Dreizen *et al.*, 1952; Grad, 1952; Warming-Larsen *et al.*, 1952). Concentrations of plasma cortisol are lowest in the early morning before wakening and reach a peak by about mid-day (Shuster, 1961). It would seem reasonable to infer from these data that the salivary $Na^+ : K^+$ ratio varies inversely with the plasma cortisol level, and the intense histochemical utilization of cortisol by the salivary duct indicates the probable site of this controlling mechanism.

The rationale of the varying salivary excretion of sodium and potassium is obscure, although an analogous corticosteroid controlled system exists in birds and reptiles in the form of the salt gland (Holmes, 1965).

II. INTESTINAL TRACT

Few accounts exist in the literature of histochemical localization of hydroxysteroid dehydrogenases in the alimentary tract. Pearson and Grose (1959) noted 17β-hydroxysteroid dehydrogenase in mouse gut, and Baillie *et al.* (1966) recorded the presence of 17β-hydroxysteroid dehydrogenase in the mucosa of the human small intestine, and particularly in human duodenal mucosa. In this laboratory these early observations have been extended in two principal ways. First, an extended phylogenetic survey of the entire alimentary tract for 3α-, 3β-, 6β-, 11β-, 12α-, 16α-, 16β-, 17α-, 17β-, 20α-, 20β-, 21- and 24-hydroxysteroid dehydrogenases has been undertaken and the unpublished data are summarized in Table 18. Secondly, the distribution of 17β-hydroxysteroid dehydrogenase in the human duodenal, jejunal and ileal mucosa recorded by Baillie *et al.* (1966) has been investigated much more fully with respect to age and sex distribution and substrate specificity.

TABLE 18

Species survey of histochemical utilization of 3α-, 3β-, 6β-, 11β-, 12α-, 16α-, 16β-, 17α-, 17β-, 20α-, 20β-, 21- and 24-hydroxysteroids by the alimentary canal

Animal	Enzyme present	Site
Goldfish	—	—
Rana Temporaria	—	—
Tortoise	—	—
Cat	17β-Hydroxysteroid dehydrogenase	Duodenal mucosa
Dog	17β-Hydroxysteroid dehydrogenase	Duodenal mucosa
Hamster	—	
Monkey	17β-Hydroxysteroid dehydrogenase	Duodenal mucosa
Mouse	17β-Hydroxysteroid dehydrogenase	Small intestinal mucosa
Rat	17β-Hydroxysteroid dehydrogenase	Duodenal mucosa

Appraisal of Table 18 indicates that in fish, amphibian and reptilian alimentary tracts no histochemically detectable hydroxysteroid dehydrogenase activity exists in any region. In the mammalian alimentary tract, *on balance*, 17β-hydroxysteroid dehydrogenase seems to be more or less consistently present in small intestinal mucosa; but we must stress that the reaction is much weaker than that seen in the human duodenal mucosa, and we have encountered persistent difficulties with positive controls. In these circumstances we feel that re-investigation of the alimentary tracts of lower mammals with biochemical methods is desirable to confirm what must be regarded as a *tentative* histochemical conclusion.

By contrast, Goldman *et al.* (1965) record strong 17β-hydroxysteroid dehydrogenase activity with testosterone and oestradiol in rat gut and do not seem to have encountered control problems (Baillie *et al.*, 1966).

In the human alimentary tract the situation is very much clearer. Positive controls have rarely been encountered, and no 3α-, 3β-, 6β-, 11β-, 16α-, 16β-, 20α-, 20β-, 21- or 24-hydroxysteroid dehydrogenase activity has been seen in stomach, duodenum, jejunum, ileum, colon or rectum.

12α-Hydroxyprogesterone gives no colour reaction with sections of stomach, duodenum or jejunum (Baillie *et al.*, 1966), but a very weak reaction can be detected in the surface epithelium of the ileum and colon, monoformazan only being deposited. Steroids with a 12α-hydroxyl group belong to the class of the bile acids and in mammalian species cholic (3α-,7α-,12α-trihydroxy-5β-cholanic, acid), and deoxycholic (3α,12α-dihydroxy-5β-cholanic acid)

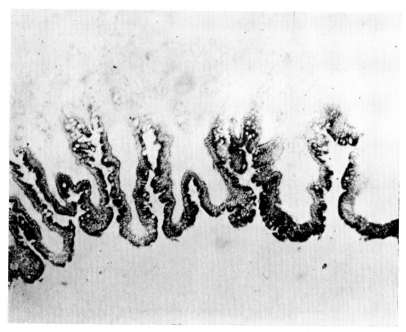

FIG. 77. Intense 17β-hydroxysteroid dehydrogenase activity in the human duodenal mucosa, using testosterone as substrate. × 100.

chenodeoxycholic (3α,7α-dihydroxy-5β-cholanic acid) acids are the most important secreted in the bile (Danielsson, 1963). 12-Ketocholanic acids have been isolated from faeces (Norman and Sjovall, 1958; Danielsson *et al.*, 1963). Since these degradation products can only be isolated from faeces, and not from fistular bile, it can be inferred that 12α-hydroxysteroid dehydrogenase is present in the alimentary canal distal to the entry of the bile duct, or in its bacterial flora. Danielsson (1963) considered that 12α-dehydrogenation was most probably the result of microbial activity in the gut, and the extremely weak 12α-hydroxysteroid dehydrogenase activity in colonic mucosa would appear to corroborate this.

The principal histochemical finding in the gut studies has been the establishment of the presence of a 17β-hydroxysteroid dehydrogenase in the mucosa of the human duodenum (Fig. 77), and, to a lesser extent, jejunum and ileum.

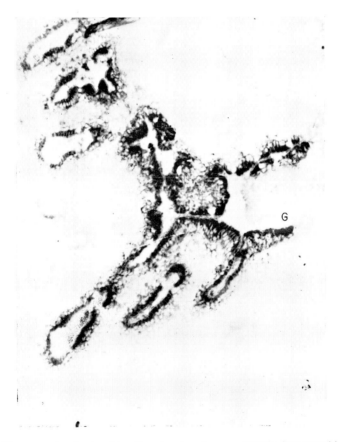

FIG. 78. Human gastro-duodenal junction showing absence of 17β-hydroxysteroid dehydrogenase in gastric mucosa (G) and intense reactivity in duodenal mucosa. The boundary line is sharp and clear-cut. Oestradiol was the substrate employed. × 40.

There is no trace of 17β-hydroxysteroid dehydrogenase activity in human gastric or colonic mucosa, and the transition from negative gastric mucosa to intense 17β-hydroxysteroid dehydrogenase activity in duodenal mucosa at the gastroduodenal junction (Fig. 78) is abrupt and striking. Another interesting anatomical feature is that ectopic intestinal mucosa in the stomach is selectively picked out on account of its intense 17β-hydroxysteroid dehydrogenase activity (Fig. 79), which contrasts with the unreactive surrounding gastric mucosa. Such islets of reactive ectopic intestinal mucosa can be recog-

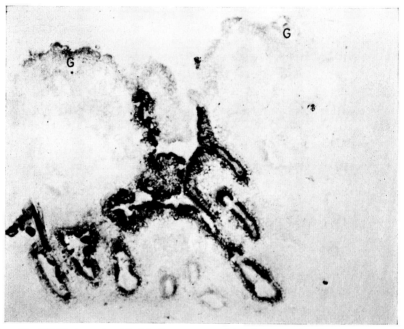

FIG. 79. 17β-Hydroxysteroid dehydrogenase activity in a patch of ectopic intestinal epithelium lying, deeply placed, in unreactive gastric (G) mucosa. Testosterone propionate was used as substrate. × 135.

nized even on naked-eye inspection of sections of gastric mucosa as blue pin-points in the uncoloured tissue.

The age distribution of human duodenal 17β-hydroxysteroid dehydrogenase is not yet fully established. In six foetuses, ranging in length from 14 mm to 23 cm, no histochemically demonstrable 17β-hydroxysteroid dehydrogenase was found (A. H. Baillie, M. M. Ferguson and D. McK. Hart, unpublished observations). 17β-Hydroxysteroid dehydrogenase was constantly present in duodenal biopsies from 20 patients ranging in age from 26 to 70 years; no obvious age or sex differences occurred in the material surveyed by this laboratory. From this it will be seen that it remains to be ascertained at which point in development 17β-hydroxysteroid dehydrogenase becomes histochemically present in duodenal mucosa. The final point to be made in connection with the anatomical distribution of 17β-hydroxysteroid dehydrogenase in the human small intestine is that the reaction is most intense in the first part of the duodenum and diminishes progressively as one examines biopsies from more distal areas such as the jejunum and ileum.

The substrate-specificity of human duodenal 17β-hydroxysteroid dehydrogenase was investigated by Baillie *et al.* (1966) on a limited number of biopsies. The number of biopsies investigated has been greatly increased, as have the range of substrates handled and the available data on the substrate-specificity of human duodenal 17β-hydroxysteroid dehydrogenase are summarized in Table 19.

TABLE 19

Substrate specificity of human small intestinal 17β-hydroxysteroid dehydrogenase

Testosterone	+ + +	17β-Hydroxy-5α-androstan-3-one	+ +
Testosterone propionate	+ + +	17β-Hydroxy-5β-androstan-3-one	trace
Testosterone phenylpropionate	+ + +	5α-Androstan-3, 17-dione	−
Testosterone isocaproate	+	5β-Androstan-3, 17-dione	−
Testosterone decanoate	trace	Androstenediol	+ + +
Testosterone sulphate	−	Oestradiol-17β	+ + +
Nortestosterone	+ +	Epitestosterone	−
Methyl testosterone	−	Epioestradiol	−
		17α-Hydroxyprogesterone	−

From the results noted in Table 19 a number of conclusions can be drawn regarding the substrate-specificity of duodenal 17β-hydroxysteroid dehydrogenase, subject to the proviso that solubility factors and membrane-permeability effects cannot be wholly excluded.

(1) Human duodenal 17β-hydroxysteroid dehydrogenase is specific for 17β-hydroxysteroids and is unable to dehydrogenate 17α-hydroxysteroids.

(2) Aromatic, Δ^4-3-keto and Δ^5-3β-hydroxy A-ring configurations are more or less equally well utilized, and the enzyme appears to be relatively indifferent to A-ring configuration. Steroids with a saturated A-ring, however, are less well utilized; in particular the 5β-configuration appears to seriously interfere with enzyme-substrate binding. Since the androstan-diketones themselves give no colour, the reaction with 17β-hydroxy-5α-androstan-3-one can probably be attributed entirely to 17β-hydroxysteroid dehydrogenase action.

(3) The unusual A-ring configuration of nortestosterone does not markedly interfere with enzyme-substrate binding.

(4) The presence of a 17α-methyl group totally obstructs 17β-dehydrogenation.

(5) The utilization of a number of testosterone esters may point to the existence of an esterase in close relationship with the dehydrogenase, but other interpretations of these observations are possible.

Baillie *et al.* (1966) considered that the aromatic A-ring, characteristic of the oestrogens, was more reactive than other A-ring configurations, but this impression has not been confirmed by the extensive follow-up studies undertaken. From the above histochemical results it is not possible to ascertain the physiological substrate for duodenal 17β-hydroxysteroid dehydrogenase.

The utilization of androstenediol by the duodenal mucosa might suggest the presence of a mucosal 3β-hydroxysteroid dehydrogenase, but no other 3β-hydroxysteroids give a colour reaction with this tissue. In these circumstances it seems reasonable to infer that the colour observed with androstenediol is due to dehydrogenation of the 17β- rather than the 3β-hydroxyl group.

The interpretation to be placed on human duodenal 17β-hydroxysteroid dehydrogenase is unclear. It may be concerned in the transfer of hydrogen between NAD- and NADP-dependent systems (Fig. 8); if such a trans-hydrogenase function were important in the cellular economy in duodenal mucosa it might explain some of the observed effects of sex hormones in duodenal ulceration and might imply that the duodenal mucosa serves as a target organ for 17β-hydroxysteroids. In this connection several clinical observations are of direct interest.

Duodenal ulceration is seldom seen in women during their reproductive years, and the fact that duodenal ulcers usually heal and seldom bleed or perforate during pregnancy suggests that female endocrines may play a part in the prevention of peptic ulceration (Johnston, 1965). Winkelstein (1936) noted that oestrogens accelerated the healing of experimental peptic ulcers in dogs, and found some indication that oestrogens were of clinical benefit to patients with duodenal ulceration. Similarly, Clark (1953), on the basis of clinical observations, postulated that circulating oestrogens have an 'anti-ulcer' effect, and it seems unlikely that this effect is accomplished by an oestrogen-induced reduction in gastric acid secretion (Clark and Tankel, 1954; Johnston and Parbhoo, 1965). There is thus circumstantial, but fairly convincing, evidence that oestrogens influence the stability of the duodenal mucosa, and the observed 17β-hydroxysteroid dehydrogenase in small intestinal mucosa may or may not be related to this finding.

Another possible function for duodenal 17β-hydroxysteroid dehydrogenase is steroid inactivation and excretion. In this connection it is interesting to note that Diczfalusy *et al.* (1961, 1962) have shown that the human intestine can dehydrogenate oestradiol-17β to oestrone and convert oestriol, oestradiol-17β and oestrone to the corresponding glucuronoside or glucosiduronate.

REFERENCES

Baillie, A. H., Calman, K. C. and MacKay, C. (1966). The histochemical distribution of hydroxysteroid dehydrogenases in human alimentary tract. *J. Roy. Microscop. Soc.* **85**, 45–52.
Clark, D. H. (1953). Peptic ulcer in women. *Brit. Med. J.* **i**, 1254–1257.

Clark, D. H. and Tankel, H. I. (1954). Gastric acid and plasma-histamine during pregnancy. *Lancet* **ii**, 886–887.

Danielsson, H. (1963). In: *Advances in Lipid Research* Vol. 1, p. 335 (Academic Press, London).

Danielsson, H., Eneroth, D., Hellstrom, K., Linstedt, S. and Sjovall, T. (1963). On the turnover and excretory products of cholic and chenodeoxycholic acid in man. *J. Biol. Chem.* **238**, 2299–2304.

De Traverse, P. M. and Coquelet, M.-L. (1952). Variations nycthémérales du rappart sodium/potassium dans la salive et l'urine. *Compt. Rend. Soc. Biol.* **146**, 1099–1102.

Diczfalusy, E., Franksson, C. and Martinsen, B. (1961). Oestrogen conjugation by the human intestinal tract. *Acta Endocrinol.* **38**, 59–72.

Diczfalusy, E., Franksson, C., Lisboa, B. A. and Martinsen, B. (1962). Formation of oestrone glucosiduronate by the human intestinal tract. *Acta Endocrinol.* **40**, 537–551.

Dreizen, S., Niedermeier, W., Reed, A. and Spies, T. M. (1952). The effect of ACTH and cortisone on the sodium and potassium levels of human saliva. *J. Dental Res.* **31**, 271–280.

Grad, B. (1951). Diurnal and age changes in the sodium and potassium concentration of human mixed saliva. *J. Gerantol.* **6**, 93 (Suppl.).

Grad, B. (1952). The influence of ACTH on the sodium and potassium concentration of human mixed saliva. *J. Clin. Endocrinol.* **12**, 708–718.

Goldman, A. S., Yakovac, W. C. and Bongiovanni, A. M. (1965). Persistent effects of a synthetic androstene derivative on activities of 3β-hydroxysteroid dehydrogenase and glucose-6-phosphate dehydrogenase in rats. *Endocrinology* **77**, 1105–1118.

Holmes, W. N. (1965). Some aspects of osmoregulation in reptiles and birds. *Arch. Anat. Microscop. Morphol. Exptl.* **54**, 491–514.

Johnston, I. D. A. (1965). Reduction of gastric acid secretion without operation. In: *Recent advances in gastroenterology* (Badenoch and Brooke) (Churchill, London).

Johnston, I. D. A. and Parbhoo, S. L. (1965). Unpublished data. Quoted by Johnstone (1965).

Maximow, A. N. and Bloom, W. (1942). *Text book of histology* pp. 365–373. (Saunders, Philadelphia).

Norman, A. and Sjovall, J. (1958). On the transformation and enterohepatic circulation of cholic acid in the rat. *J. Biol. Chem.* **233**, 872–885.

Pearson, B. and Grose, F. (1959). Histochemical demonstration of 17β-hydroxysteroid dehydrogenase by use of tetrazolium salt. *Proc. Soc. Exptl. Biol. Med.* **100**, 636–638.

Shuster, S. (1961). Quoted by Bell, G. H., Davidson, J. M. and Scarborough, H. (1961). *Textbook of Physiology and Biochemistry* Ch. 51, p. 976 (Livingstone, Edinburgh).

Warming-Larsen, A., Hamburger, C. and Sprechler, M. (1952). The influence of ACTH on the sodium and potassium concentration of human saliva. *Acta Endocrinol.* **11**, 400–412.

Winkelstein, A. (1936). Observations on ulceration adjacent to experimental gastric pouches in dogs. *Am. J. Digest. Diseases* **3**, 229–231.

CHAPTER 9

The Liver

Biochemical and clinical studies have clearly shown that the liver is extensively involved in steroid metabolism. From the histochemical standpoint it is unusual in several respects. First, it is more difficult to control than most other tissues, the main reason being probably its intrinsic content of substrates such as succinate, malate, etc., which are potential hydrogen sources, together with their appropriate dehydrogenases. Secondly, the tissue is homogeneous to an extent not found in other organs dealt with in this book. In consequence, the histological distribution of hydroxysteroid dehydrogenases in the liver can be dismissed briefly with the comment that they are confined to the liver cells proper and do not occur to any extent in the sinus endothelium or bile duct epithelium. Moreover, we have seen little evidence of any zonal differences in activity (see Figs. 80–82) within the hepatic lobule. As a result of this homogeneous distribution of hydroxysteroid dehydrogenase activity, the results of comparative incubations (Fig. 83) can

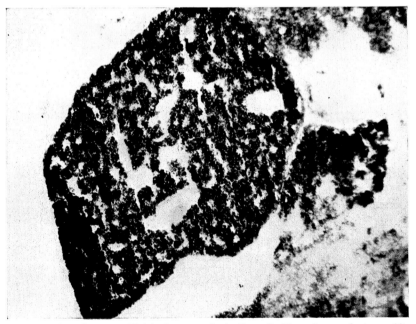

FIG. 80. 17β-Hydroxysteroid dehydrogenase in the liver of a 14 mm human foetus. × 80.

almost be judged by the naked eye; more important, this is one tissue where quantitation of hydroxysteroid dehydrogenase activity could be undertaken using light absorption techniques, although this has not yet been attempted.

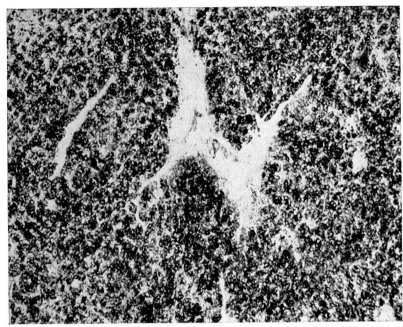

Fig. 81. 3α-Hydroxysteroid dehydrogenase in the adult cockerel liver. Note the even distribution of the reaction product in the hepatic tissue. × 60.

Our knowledge of the species and sex distribution of hepatic hydroxysteroid dehydrogenase activity is summarized in Table 20. The available data relating to foetal and adult human liver are listed in Table 21. The remainder of this chapter will be devoted to relating the histochemical observations to what is

TABLE 21

Distribution of hydroxysteroid dehydrogenase in human liver (Baillie *et al.* 1966, and unpublished)

Source	Type of hydroxysteroid dehydrogenase							
	3α	Δ^5-3β	6β	11β	16α	16β	17β	20β
14 mm foetus	trace	−	−	−	+	−	+ +	−
12–24 cm foetuses	+	+ poor	−	−	trace	+	+ +	−
Adult (male)	+	trace	trace	+	+	+	+ +	−
Adult (female)	+	trace	−	+	+	+	+ +	−

TABLE 20

Species and sex distribution of hepatic hydroxysteroid dehydrogenase

Animal	3α	Δ^5-3β	6β	11β	16α	16β	17β	20β	Investigator
				Type of hydroxysteroid dehydrogenase					
Goldfish	++	+	trace	−	+	+	+	−	Unpublished data
Rana temporaria	+	−	−	−	+	+	+	−	Unpublished data
Tortoise	+++	−	−	−	+	+	+	−	Unpublished data
Cockerel	++	+	+	+	+++	+++	++	−	Unpublished data
Dog (female)	++	trace	−	+	+	++	++	−	Unpublished data
Guinea-pig (male)	+	+	trace	−	+	+	+	trace	Baillie et al. (1966)
Guinea-pig (female)	+	+	trace	trace	trace	+	+	trace	Baillie et al. (1966)
Hamster (male)	+	+	+	+	+	+	+	trace	Baillie et al. (1966)
Hamster (female)	+	+	trace	+	+	trace	+	trace	Baillie et al. (1966)
Mouse (male)	+	trace	trace	+	+	+	+	trace	Baillie et al. (1966)
Mouse (female)	+	trace	trace	+	trace	trace	+	trace	Baillie et al. (1966)
Rat (male)	+	+	trace	+	+	+	+	trace	Baillie et al. (1966)
Rat (female)	+	trace	trace	trace	trace	trace	+	trace	Baillie (et al. 1966)

known of the biochemical features of hepatic hydroxysteroid dehydrogenases.

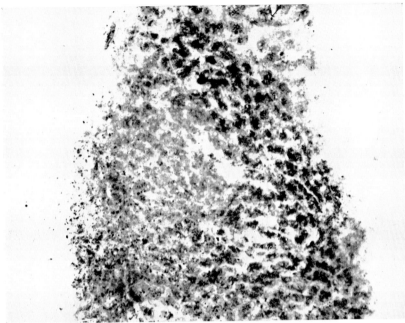

FIG. 82. 17β-Hydroxysteroid dehydrogenase in adult human liver tissue obtained by needle biopsy for diagnostic purposes. × 70.

A. 3α-HYDROXYSTEROID DEHYDROGENASE

Pearson and Grose (1959a) were the first to note histochemically hepatic 3α-hydroxysteroid dehydrogenase, although no species was quoted. The extensive species distribution noted in Table 20 was established in this laboratory (Baillie *et al.*, 1966, and unpublished observations), and could have been foreseen from biochemical work (Schneider and Mason, 1948a, b; Ungar and Dorfman, 1954; Tomkins, 1956; Rubin, 1957; Benard *et al.*, 1961).

Hepatic 3α-hydroxysteroid dehydrogenase (Fig. 21) is thought to be concerned with the detoxication and excretion of steroids; it interconverts 3-ketosteroids, such as androstenedione, with 3α-hydroxysteroids, such as androsterone and aetiocholanolone (Vande Wiele *et al.*, 1963), a reductase also being involved. Conjugation and excretion then follow (Tomkins and Isselbacher, 1954). Tomkins (1956) found biochemically that both 5α- and 5β-steroisomers were suitable substrates for 3α-hydroxysteroid dehydrogenase, but histochemically the 5α-isomer is usually better utilized than the 5β-isomer. In this connection it is interesting to note that clinically aetiocholanolone (a 3α-hydroxy 5β-steroid) gives rise to pyrexia whereas the corresponding 3α-hydroxy 5α-steroid does not (Kappas *et al.*, 1958); more-

Control

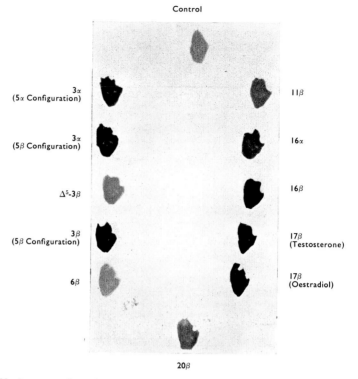

3α
(5α Configuration)

3α
(5β Configuration)

Δ⁵-3β

3β
(5β Configuration)

6β

11β

16α

16β

17β
(Testosterone)

17β
(Oestradiol)

20β

FIG. 83. A group of rat liver sections after incubation, showing the relative intensity of different hydrosysteroid dehydrogenase reactions. × ½.

over, in aetiocholanolone fever most of the injected steroid is excreted unchanged in the urine.

Both biochemically (Hurlock and Talalay, 1958; Koide, 1963; Aoshima *et al.*, 1964) and histochemically, hepatic 3α-hydroxysteroid dehydrogenase utilizes NAD and NADP as co-factor.

B. 3β-HYDROXYSTEROID DEHYDROGENASE

Using Δ⁵-3β-hydroxysteroids (Wattenberg, 1958; Baillie *et al.*, 1966; Table 20) such as pregnenolone and DHA, only poor hepatic Δ⁵-3β-hydroxysteroid dehydrogenase can be detected histochemically. In fact Goldman *et al.* (1965) failed to demonstrate this enzyme in rat liver. It is of interest that the sex differences in the biochemical distribution of 3β-hydroxysteroid dehydro- genase (Rubin, 1957; Rubin and Strecker, 1961; Rubin and Kopf, 1963) in rat liver can also be confirmed histochemically (Table 20). With 3β-hydroxy- 5β-steroids intense 3β-hydroxysteroid dehydrogenase is demonstrable in liver.

C. 6β-HYDROXYSTEROID DEHYDROGENASE

This is unconvincing histochemically in the liver. It has been described biochemically (Breuer and Pangels, 1962) in rat liver. The disparity between the biochemical and histochemical observations may be attributed to differences in the thresholds involved in the two techniques. The hepatic enzyme may be concerned in steroid excretion, and Lipman et al. (1962) have suggested that 6β-hydroxy derivatives of cortisol are more soluble polar steroids and more suitable for excretion.

D. 11β-HYDROXYSTEROID DEHYDROGENASE

Biochemical evidence for the existence of hepatic 11β-hydroxysteroid dehydrogenase exists in rat, bovine, porcine and human liver (Eisenstein, 1952; Caspi et al., 1953; Fish et al., 1953; Caspi and Hechter, 1954; Caspi, 1955; Meigs and Engel, 1961). Koerner and Hellman (1964) noted sex differences in NAD- and NADP-linked 11β-hydroxysteroid dehydrogenase in rat liver, and these have been noted histochemically. The precise biochemical role of hepatic 11β-hydroxysteroid dehydrogenase is uncertain, and it may be involved in either corticosteroid or androgen metabolism.

E. 16α-HYDROXYSTEROID DEHYDROGENASE

This enzyme occurs histochemically in a wide variety of livers (Table 20), and there is a biochemical precedent for these observations in human, rat and guinea-pig liver (Breuer et al., 1958, 1959; Correale and Balestreri, 1962). The enzyme may be concerned with oestrogen metabolism in the liver (Fig. 53), but this supposition at present lacks proof.

F. 16β-HYDROXYSTEROID DEHYDROGENASE

This enzyme is extremely active in avian liver histochemically but is not strong (Table 20) in mammalian liver, notwithstanding the biochemical findings of Breuer and Knuppen (1958). Sex differences occur histochemically but the significance of these observations cannot be commented on until more is known of the biochemical role of this enzyme.

G. 17β-HYDROXYSTEROID DEHYDROGENASE

17β-Hydroxysteroid dehydrogenase activity has been noted biochemically in foetal and adult human (Stylianou et al., 1961; Engel et al., 1958), mouse, rat, rabbit, hamster and dog livers (Endahl et al., 1960; Villee and Spencer, 1960; Endahl and Kochakian, 1962; Aoshima and Kochakian, 1963; El Attar et al., 1964). Histochemically it was first noted in rat liver (Pearson and Grose, 1959b) and it is extremely active in human foetal liver (Fig. 80). It is present (Table 21) before the adult pattern of hydroxysteroid dehydrogenase activity appears. In view of the involvement of this enzyme in androgen and oestrogen metabolism this observation is of particular interest in that it suggests that specific ability to metabolize sex steroids may be acquired by the foetal liver in advance of its more general steroid metabolic pathways.

The substrate specificity of human hepatic 17β-hydroxysteroid dehydrogenase in a histochemical system is indicated in Table 22.

TABLE 22

Histochemical utilization of 17-hydroxysteroids by human liver tissue

Testosterone	+ +	17β-Hydroxy-5α-androstan-3-one	+
Testosterone propionate	+ +	17β-Hydroxy-5β-androstan-3-one	–
Testosterone phenyl propionate	+ +	Oestradiol-17β	+ +
Testosterone isocaproate	+ +	Epitestosterone	–
Testosterone decanoate	+	17α-Hydroxyprogesterone	–
Testosterone sulphate	–		

H. 20α-HYDROXYSTEROID DEHYDROGENASE

This enzyme has been demonstrated biochemically in pig (Caspi *et al.*, 1956), and rabbit (Taylor, 1959) liver. Balogh (1964) failed histochemically to detect this enzyme in rat liver, and we can find no other references to it in the histochemical literature.

I. 20β-HYDROXYSTEROID DEHYDROGENASE

20β-Hydroxysteroid dehydrogenase activity is extremely disappointing (Table 20) histochemically, although it has been established biochemically in rat liver (Caspi *et al.*, 1953; Caspi and Hechter, 1954; Caspi, 1955).

11α-, 17α-, 21- and 24-hydroxysteroids are not used to any extent by any liver tissue surveyed in this laboratory. NAD-linked ovine, bovine and porcine hepatic 21-hydroxysteroid dehydrogenase occurs (Mander and White, 1963), but the equilibrium appears to strongly favour reduction; this might account for the histochemical absence of demonstrable hepatic 21-hydroxysteroid dehydrogenase.

In conclusion, the histochemical findings with liver tissue are of principally biochemical interest. The uniformity of the tissue is such that the activity of given hydroxysteroid dehydrogenases can be directly and readily compared. Given stable section thickness, this rough quantitation can readily be refined and reaction intensity measured easily by virtue of differences in light absorption. The technique would lend itself, in these circumstances, to a study of factors influencing hydroxysteroid dehydrogenase activity and could prove a useful screening technique in a biochemical study. Of embryological interest is the fact that human yolk-sac, small intestine and liver all possess 17β-hydroxysteroid dehydrogenase in their endodermal components. Moreover, we have noted a weak 17β-hydroxysteroid dehydrogenase reaction in murine gall bladder epithelium. The histochemical similarity between these four tissues is intriguing in view of their common developmental origin.

REFERENCES

Aoshima, Y. and Kochakian, C. D. (1963). Activity, intracellular distribution and some properties of 17β-hydroxy-C-19-steroid dehydrogenases in liver and kidney. *Endocrinology* **72**, 106–114.

Aoshima, Y., Kochakian, C. D. and Jadrijevic, D. (1964). TPN and DPN-specific 3α-hydroxy and Δ^5-3β-hydroxysteroid dehydrogenases of liver and kidney. *Endocrinology* **74**, 521–531.

Baillie, A. H., Calman, K. C., Ferguson, M. M. and Hart, D. McK. (1966). Histochemical distribution of hydroxysteroid dehydrogenases in kidney and liver. *Histochemie* **5**, 384–395.

Balogh, K. (1964). A histochemical method for the demonstration of 20α-hydroxysteroid dehydrogenase activity in rat ovaries. *J. Histochem. Cytochem.* **12**, 670–673.

Benard, H., Cruz-Horn, A. and David, H. (1961). Sur le mecanisme de la transformation de l'androsterone et de l'epiandrosterone au cours de la perfusion du foie isole de Lapin, en aerobiose. *Compt. Rend. Soc. Biol.* **155**, 235.

Breuer, H. and Knuppen, R. (1958). Metabolism of 16-oxo-oestrone by human liver slices *in vitro*. *Nature* **182**, 1512.

Breuer, H. and Pangels, G. (1962). Konfiguration, Biogenese und Stoffwechsel von 6α- und 6β-hydroxylierten phenolischen steroiden. *Biochim. Biophys. Acta* **65**, 1–12.

Breuer, H., Knuppen, R. and Pangels, G. (1962). Konfiguration, Biogenese und Stoffwechsel von 16α- and 16β-hydroxylierten phenolischen steroiden. *Biochim. Biophys. Acta* **65**, 1–12.

Breuer, H., Nocke, L. and Knuppen, R. (1958). Reduktion von 16α-hydroxyoestron und 16-keto-oestradiol-(17β) durch menschliches Lebergewebe *in vitro*. *Z. Physiol. Chem.* **311**, 275–278.

Breuer, H., Nocke, L. and Knuppen, R. (1959). Metabolic reduction of 16α-hydroxyoestrone and 16-oxooestradiol-17β by liver tissue *in vitro*. *Biochim. Biophys. Acta* **33**, 254–256.

Caspi, E. (1955). Ph.D. Thesis. Clark University, Worcester, Mass., U.S.A. (Quoted by Dorfman and Ungar (1965)).

Caspi, E. and Hechter, O. (1954). Corticosteroid metabolism in liver. III. Isolation of additional cortisone metabolites. *Arch. Biochem. Biophys.* **52**, 478–483.

Caspi, E., Levy, H. and Hechter, O. (1953). Cortisone metabolism in liver. II. Isolation of certain cortisone metabolites. *Arch. Biochem. Biophys.* **45**, 169–182.

Caspi, E., Lindberg, M. C., Hayano, M., Cohen, J. L., Matsuba, M., Rosenkrantz, H. and Dorfman, R. I. (1956). The C-20 reduction of steroids by hog liver preparations. *Arch. Biochem. Biophys.* **61**, 267–271.

Correale, L. and Balestreri, R. (1962). Metabolism of oestrogens oxygenated in position C-16. Conversion *in vitro* of estriol-16-keto to 17β-oestradiol by rat liver. *Arch. Maragliano Patol. Clin.* **18**, 653–658.

Eisenstein, A. B. (1952). Steroid compounds resulting from incubation of cortisone with surviving liver slices. *Science* **116**, 520–521.

El Attar, T., Mosebach, K. O. and Dirscherl, W. (1964). The initial metabolism of 4-^{14}C-testosterone in the rat. II. In liver, blood plasma, seminal vesicles and ventral prostate. *Acta Endocrinol.* **45**, 437–446.

Endahl, G. L. and Kochakian, C. D. (1962). Partial purification and further characterization of the triphosphopyridine nucleotide specific C19-17β-hydroxysteroid dehydrogenase of guinea-pig liver. *Biochim. Biophys. Acta* **62**, 245–250.

Endahl, G. L., Kochakian, C. D. and Hamm, D. (1960). Separation of a TPN-specific from a DPN-specific 17β-hydroxy (testosterone) dehydrogenase of guinea-pig liver. *J. Biol. Chem.* **235**, 2792–2796.

Engel, L. L., Baggett, B. and Halla, M. (1958). The formation of ¹⁴C-labelled estriol from 16-¹⁴C-estradiol-17β by human fetal liver slices. *Biochim. Biophys. Acta* **30**, 435–436.

Fish, C. A., Hayano, M. and Pincus, G. (1953). Conversion of cortisone to 17-hydroxycorticosterone by liver homogenates. *Arch. Biochem. Biophys.* **42**, 480–481.

Goldman, A. S., Yakovac, W. C. and Bongiovanni, A. M. (1965). Persistent effects of a synthetic androstene derivative on activities of 3β-hydroxysteroid dehydrogenase and glucose-6-phosphate dehydrogenase in rats. *Endocrinology* **77**, 1105–1118.

Hurlock, B. and Talalay, P. (1958). 3α-hydroxysteroids as co-enzymes of hydrogen transfer between di- and tri-phosphopyridine nucleotides. *J. Biol. Chem.* **233**, 886–897.

Kappas, A., Soybel, W., Fukushima, D. I. K. and Gallagher, T. F. (1958). The thermogenic effect and metabolic fate of etiocholanolone in man. *J. Clin. Endocrinol.* **18**, 1043–1055.

Koerner, D. R. and Hellman, L. (1964). Effect of thyroxine administration on the 11β-hydroxysteroid dehydrogenase in rat liver and kidney. *Endocrinology* **75**, 592–601.

Koide, S. S. (1963). Purification of 3α-hydroxysteroid dehydrogenase obtained from the soluble fraction of rat liver. *Arch. Biochem.* **101**, 278–285.

Lipman, M. M., Katz, F. H. and Jailer, J. W. (1962). An alternate pathway for cortisol metabolism 6β-hydroxy cortisol production by human tissue slices. *J. Clin. Endocrinol.* **22**, 268–272.

Mander, C. and White, A. (1963). Purification and properties of a sheep liver 21-hydroxysteroid-NAD-oxido reductase. *J. Biol. Chem.* **238**, 767–774.

Meigs, R. A. and Engel, L. L. (1961). The metabolism of adrenocortical steroids by human tissues. *Endocrinology* **69**, 152–162.

Pearson, B. and Grose, F. (1959a). Histochemical study of some DPNH and DPN dependent dehydrogenases. *Federation Proc.* **18**, 499.

Pearson, B. and Grose, F. (1959b). Histochemical demonstration of 17β-hydroxysteroid dehydrogenase by use of tetrazolium salt. *Proc. Soc. Exptl. Biol. Med.* **100**, 636–638.

Rubin, B. L. (1957). Sex differences in orientation of reduction products of 3-keto, C¹⁹ steroids by rat liver homogenates. *J. Biol. Chem.* **227**, 917–927.

Rubin, B. L. and Kopf, E. B. (1963). Further observations on sex-influenced activity of 3β-hydroxysteroid dehydrogenase of rat liver. *Endocrinology* **72**, 764–770.

Rubin, B. L. and Strecker, H. J. (1961). Further studies on the sex difference in 3β-hydroxysteroid dehydrogenase activity of rat livers. *Endocrinology* **69**, 257–267.

Schneider, J. J. and Mason, H. L. (1948a). Studies on intermediary steroid metabolism. I. *J. Biol. Chem.* **172**, 771–782.

Schneider, J. J. and Mason, H. L. (1948b). Studies on intermediary steroid metabolism II. *J. Biol. Chem.* **175**, 231–240.

Stylianou, M., Forchielli, E., Tummillo, M. and Dorfman, R. I. (1961). Metabolism *in vitro* of 4-C¹⁴-testosterone by a human liver homogenate. *J. Biol. Chem.* **236**, 629–694.

Taylor, W. (1959). Investigation of the products of metabolism after incubation of deoxycorticosterone with rabbit liver homogenate. *Biochem. J.* **72**, 442–450.

Tomkins, G. M. (1956). A mammalian 3α-hydroxysteroid dehydrogenase. *J. Biol. Chem.* **218**, 437–447.

Tomkins, G. M. and Isselbacher, K. J. (1954). Enzymic reduction of cortisone. *J. Am. Chem. Soc.* **76**, 3100–3101.

Ungar, F. and Dorfman, R. I. (1954). The conversion of 17α-, 21-dihydroxypregnane-3, 20-dione to 3α, 17α, 21-trihydroxypregnan-20-one. *J. Am. Chem. Soc.* **76**, 1197–1198.

Vande Wiele, R. L., MacDonald, P. C., Gurpide, E. and Lieberman, S. (1963). Studies on the secretion and interconversion of the androgens. *Recent Progr. Hormone Res.* **19**, 275–310.

Villee, C. A. and Spencer, J. M. (1960). Some properties of the pyridine nucleotide-specific 17β-hydroxysteroid dehydrogenases of guinea-pig liver. *J. Biol. Chem.* **235**, 3615–3619.

Wattenberg, L. W. (1958). Microscopic histochemical demonstration of steroid-3β-ol dehydrogenase in tissue sections. *J. Histochem. Cytochem.* **6**, 225–232.

CHAPTER 10

The Placenta, Hydatidiform Moles, Foetal Membranes and Yolk Sac

I. The Placenta

Progesterone, oestradiol-17β and various metabolites have been isolated from placental tissue, and an increasing number of related steroids have been isolated during recent years, including 6β-, 11β- and 16α-hydroxylated compounds. The amount of steroid produced by the placenta increases gradually towards term and a maximum is reached during the ninth month, shortly before term. Actual production or secretion of corticoids and androgens by placental tissue has not been demonstrated, however; the origin of substances found in placenta from the circulatory blood, for example (Axelrod and Werthessen, 1961), cannot be discounted. With these facts in mind the histochemical distribution of placental hydroxysteroid dehydrogenases can now be considered.

A. 3α-hydroxysteroid dehydrogenase

The histochemical occurrence of 3α-hydroxysteroid dehydrogenase in the placenta is summarized in Table 23.

TABLE 23

Histochemical distribution of 3α-hydroxysteroid dehydrogenase in the placenta

Substrate	Co-factor	Species	Remarks	Investigators
Androsterone and aetiocholanolone	NAD and NADP	Human	Absent	Koide and Mitsudo (1965)
Androsterone and aetiocholanolone	NAD	Human	Present in trophoblast	Baillie *et al.* (1966)
Androsterone and aetiocholanolone	NAD	Human	Present from 6 weeks to term	Hart (1966b)

A scrutiny of Table 23 indicates that Baillie *et al.* (1966) and Hart (1966a, b, c) consistently record weak 3α-hydroxysteroid dehydrogenase in human trophoblast (Fig. 84), whereas Koide and Mitsudo (1965) failed to demonstrate the enzyme histochemically. This conflict of results is more apparent than real; Koide and Mitsudo (1965) washed their sections in 80% alcohol for ten minutes after incubation, and such treatment would remove the pink mono-

152

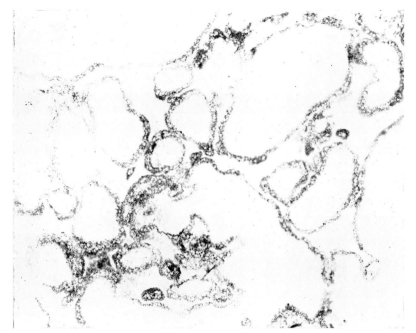

FIG. 84. 3α-Hydroxysteroid dehyrogenase activity in the trophoblast of a 6 weeks human placenta, NAD-linked. × 160.

formazan which constituted the weak reaction of other workers. The placenta can probably form urocortisol and possibly other related 3α-hydroxysteroids (Troen, 1962), but much remains to be done to elucidate the precise role of 3α-hydroxysteroid dehydrogenase in placental biochemistry.

3α-Hydroxysteroid dehydrogenase has not yet been investigated in the placentae of other mammals.

B. Δ⁵-3β-HYDROXYSTEROID DEHYDROGENASE

In his original description of human placental 3β-hydroxysteroid dehydrogenase, Wattenberg (1958) stated that it was situated in the trophoblast and was NAD-linked (Fig. 85). It is now clear that this important biosynthetic enzyme (Fig. 10) is present in the human trophoblast almost from the start of pregnancy (Table 24) and in the trophoblastic giant cells of the rodent placenta, which, according to Wislocki and Dempsey (1955), correspond to the villous syntrophoblast of the human placenta.

From Table 24 it will be seen that a wide measure of agreement exists between different investigators. The utilization (Table 24) of steroid sulphates and other esters is of particular interest. Baulieu (1960) demonstrated that plasma DHA is present mainly as its sulphate ester, and DHA sulphate has

F

been shown to constitute an oestrogen precursor in the placenta (Baulieu and Dray, 1963; Siiteri and MacDonald, 1963; Bolté *et al.*, 1964a, b, c). It appears that DHA sulphate is hydrolysed by a specific steroid sulphatase (Pulkkinen, 1961; Warren and Timberlake, 1962; Warren and French, 1965) in the human placenta before conversion of free DHA to oestrogens.

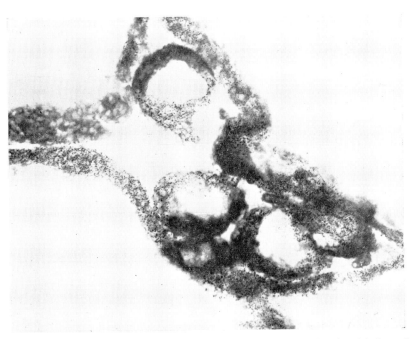

FIG. 85. NAD-linked 3β-hydroxysteroid dehydrogenase in the trophoblastic epithelium of a term human placenta. × 260.

It will be noted from Table 24 that placental 3β-hydroxysteroid dehydrogenase has dual pyridine nucleotide specificity, and this appears to be the first record of NADP-dependent 3β-hydroxysteroid dehydrogenase in human tissue.

Schiebler and Knoop (1959) distinguished two types of giant cells in electron micrographs of rat placenta but these authors and Deane *et al.* (1962) were unable to distinguish both types with the light microscope. Botte *et al.* (1966) described two generations of giant cells on the basis of time of appearance in their histochemical study of rat placenta using the light microscope. On morphological grounds Schiebler and Knoop (1959) tentatively suggested steroid hormone secretion by rat placenta trophoblastic giant cells. The presence of 3β-hydroxysteroid dehydrogenase supports such a suggestion and accords well with the supposed phylogenetic relationship between these cells and the human villous syncytiotrophoblast referred to above.

TABLE 24

Demonstration of 3β- and of Δ^5-3β-hydroxysteroid dehydrogenase in placenta

Substrate	Co-factor	Species	Remarks	Investigators
DHA and pregnenolone	NAD	Human	In trophoblast	Wattenberg (1958)
DHA	NAD	Human	In trophoblast	Fuhrmann (1961)
DHA	NAD	Rat and Mouse	Trophoblastic giant cells	Deane et al. (1962)
DHA	NAD	Human	Age distribution established	Lobel et al. (1962)
DHA	NAD	Human	Present in term and a 5 weeks placenta	Goldberg et al. (1963)
Pregnenolone 17α-Hydroxypregnenolone DHA Androstenediol 16α-Hydroxypregnenolone Pregnenolone sulphate Pregnenolone acetate 17α-Hydroxypregnenolone sulphate DHA sulphate DHA acetate	NAD	Human	All substrates used to a greater or lesser extent by the trophoblast	Baillie et al. (1965a)
Pregnenolone DHA	NAD and NADP	Human	NADP gives a colour reaction; this is weaker than that observed with NAD	Koide and Mitsudo (1965)
3β-Hydroxy-5α-androstan-17-one 3β-Hydroxy-5β-androstan-17-one 3β-Hydroxyandrost-4-en-17-one 3β-Hydroxy-5α-pregnan-20-one Pregnenolone and DHA	NAD	Rat	Activity in trophoblastic giant cells maximal between the thirteenth and fifteenth days of gestation	Botte et al. (1966)
Pregnenolone and DHA	NAD and NADP	Human	Supports report of Lobel et al. (1962)	Hart (1966b)
3β-Hydroxy-5α-pregnan-20-one 3β-Hydroxy-5β-pregnan-20-one 3β-Hydroxy-5α-androstan 3β-Hydroxy-5β-androstan-17-one	NAD and NADP	Human	5α-Configuration steroids are not used to any extent. 5β-Steroids give a massive reaction with both pyridine nucleotides	D. McK. Hart (unpublished)

F2

C. 6β-HYDROXYSTEROID DEHYDROGENASE

Baillie *et al.* (1966) described weak NAD-linked 6β-hydroxysteroid dehydrogenase in term human placental trophoblast, using 6β-hydroxyprogesterone as substrate. There is biochemical evidence of a 6β-hydroxysteroid dehydrogenase in human placenta (Iwata, 1959) which interconverts the 6β-hydroxy and 6-keto forms of pregnenolone and progesterone. From a histochemical standpoint the reaction is disappointing, and Hart (1966a) recorded 6β-hydroxysteroid dehydrogenase histochemically in only half of his placental age series.

D. 11α-HYDROXYSTEROID DEHYDROGENASE

11α-Hydroxysteroid dehydrogenase is not demonstrable histochemically in immature or mature human placenta (Baillie *et al.*, 1966; Hart, 1966a).

E. 11β-HYDROXYSTEROID DEHYDROGENASE

Following the observation that term human placental homogenates transformed adrenal 11β-hydroxysteroids into 11-keto compounds, Osinski (1960) investigated the action and properties of the corresponding enzyme biochemically, using tritium-labelled cortisol, cortisone, corticosterone and 11β-hydroxyandrostenedione. Placental 11β-hydroxysteroid dehydrogenase was both NAD- and NADP-linked; activity with NAD as co-factor was only from one-half to one-third of that with NADP as co-factor, and the pH optimum of the latter activity lay between pH 8 and pH 9. The reaction was reversible in the presence of an NADP-reducing system (glucose-6-phosphate dehydrogenase) and substrate specificity was low, both C_{19} and C_{21} steroids with or without a 17-hydroxyl group in the side-chain being transformed. The foetal membranes were a particularly rich source of the enzyme.

Baillie *et al.* (1965b) and Hart (1966a) found histochemical evidence of this enzyme in immature and mature human placental trophoblast. Cortisol and corticosterone were not employed as substrates, and the results were obtained using 11β-hydroxyandrostenedione and 11β-hydroxyprogesterone. A positive reaction was obtained only with NAD as co-factor.

The physiological role of the enzyme in trophoblast is uncertain, but its presence in placenta and membranes may explain the origin of the cortisone found in normal human liquor amnii (Baird and Bush, 1960).

F. 12α-HYDROXYSTEROID DEHYDROGENASE

12α-Hydroxysteroid dehydrogenase has not been demonstrated histochemically in placenta.

G. 16α- AND 16β-HYDROXYSTEROID DEHYDROGENASES

A number of oestrogens with either 16α- or 16β-hydroxyl groups have been isolated (Levitz *et al.*, 1958; Breuer and Nocke, 1959) and it is known that these 16-hydroxy compounds can be interconverted via the 16-keto group (Levitz *et al.*, 1960), inferring the presence of 16α- and 16β-hydroxysteroid dehydrogenases. Liver, placenta and hydatidiform mole have been shown to metabolize the 16-hydroxy oestrogens (Breuer and Knuppen, 1958; Ryan, 1960; Klausner and Ryan, 1964; MacDonald and Siiteri, 1964).

Poor histochemical evidence of 16α-hydroxysteroid dehydrogenase activity in human, term placenta was reported by Baillie *et al.* (1966) using 16α-hydroxyoestrone and 16α-hydroxyprogesterone, but Hart (1966a) was unable to find convincing histochemical evidence of 16α-hydroxysteroid dehydrogenase in a large series of human placentae.

An intensely strong histochemical reaction (Fig. 86) for 16β-hydroxysteroid dehydrogenase was reported in the trophoblast of term human placenta by Baillie *et al.* (1966), and this is present in the trophoblast of normal human placenta from the sixth to the forty-second weeks of gestation (Hart, 1966a).

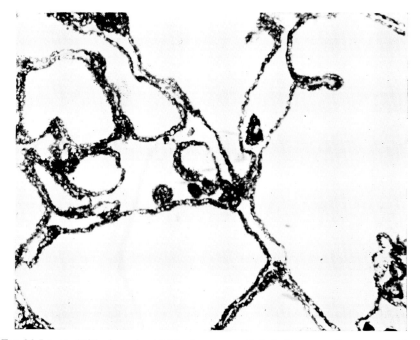

FIG. 86. Intense 16β-hydroxysteroid dehydrogenase activity in the syn- and cyto-trophoblast of a 6 weeks human placenta. × 150.

3β, 16β-Dihydroxyandrost-5-ene 3-methyl ether (with 3β-hydroxyandrost-5-en-16-one 3-methyl ether as control) and 3,16β-dihydroxyoestra-1,3,5(10)-triene were used as substrates. Both NAD and NADP are suitable co-factors, but a much stronger reaction was obtained with NAD.

The exact biochemical significance of the highly active 16β-hydroxysteroid dehydrogenase in trophoblast is not known, although from the biochemical reports cited above it would appear to be involved in oestrogen metabolism.

H. 17α-HYDROXYSTEROID DEHYDROGENASE

The 17α-hydroxyl group lies in a hindered position and is unlikely to be readily dehydrogenated. Kellogg and Glenner (1960) found no histochemical evidence of NAD- or NADP-linked 17α-hydroxysteroid dehydrogenase in term human placenta, and this accords with the findings of Baillie *et al.* (1966a) and Hart (1966a).

I. 17β-HYDROXYSTEROID DEHYDROGENASE

Ryan and Engel (1953), Levitz *et al.* (1956) and Troen (1961) have described the interconversion of oestrone and oestradiol by human tissue slices and perfused human placenta; the existence of a placental 17β-hydroxysteroid dehydrogenase is well established.

Biochemically and histochemically, placental 17β-hydroxysteroid dehydrogenase has been the subject of dispute and diversity of opinion; in particular, statements regarding the pyridine nucleotide specificity of placental oestradiol-17β dehydrogenase and its transhydrogenase function have been numerous and conflicting.

Talalay and his co-workers (Talalay *et al.*, 1958a, b) showed that soluble enzyme preparations from human placenta promoted a reversible transfer of hydrogen between pyridine nucleotides in the presence of low concentrations of 17β-hydroxysteroids or keto-steroids, especially 17β-oestradiol and oestrone. These preparations contained a 17β-hydroxysteroid dehydrogenase which interconverted 17β-oestradiol and oestrone using NAD or NADP as co-factor (Langer and Engel, 1958; Langer *et al.*, 1959), and there was close correlation between steroids which mediated the transhydrogenation function and those which underwent dehydrogenation. Jarabak *et al.* (1962) purified a soluble 17β-hydroxysteroid dehydrogenase from human placenta by an eight-step procedure resulting in an approximately 2,500-fold purification with an over-all yield of 29% and were unable to separate the dehydrogenase and transhydrogenase functions. They concluded that a soluble 17β-hydroxysteroid dehydrogenase in human placenta reacted with both NAD and NADP, and that this enzyme was responsible for most, if not all, of the 17β-oestradiol-mediated transfer of hydrogen between pyridine nucleotides.

On the other hand, Villee and his co-workers (Hagerman and Villee, 1959; Hagerman *et al.*, 1959; Villee, 1961) have claimed to have separated discrete NAD- and NADP-dependent oestradiol-17β-dehydrogenases and an oestradiol-17β-sensitive transhydrogenase.

From biochemical reports (Langer and Engel, 1958; Adams *et al.* 1962) it seems probable that oxidation of oestradiol-17β and of testosterone may be mediated by different 17β-hydroxysteroid dehydrogenases.

The histochemical accounts of placental 17β-hydroxysteroid dehydrogenase have been no less conflicting and are summarized in Table 25. In the hope of resolving the disparity revealed by Table 25, Hart (1966d) investigated the

TABLE 25

Summary of placental 17β-hydroxysteroid dehydrogenase histochemical results

Substrate	Co-factor	Distribution	Investigator
Oestradiol	NAD	Trophoblast and perivascular stroma	Kellogg and Glenner (1960)
Oestradiol	NADP	Perivascular stroma only	Kleiner *et al.* (1962)
Oestradiol	NAD	Trophoblast, stroma and blood vessels	Koide and Mitsudo (1965)
Oestradiol	NADP	Blood vessels only	
Testosterone			
17β-Hydroxy-5-androstan-3-one	NAD and NADP	Blood vessels only	
Oestriol	NAD and NADP	Not utilized	
Oestradiol	NAD	Trophoblast, stroma and blood vessels	Hart (1966a, d)
Oestradiol	NADP	Trophoblast only	
Testosterone	NAD	Blood vessels only	
Testosterone	NADP	No reaction	

distribution of placental diaphorases and noted that NAD diaphorase occurs in the trophoblast, stroma and blood vessels, whereas NADP diaphorase is largely restricted to the trophoblast. Although Hart (1966d) and Kellogg and Glenner (1960) agree that Nitro BT is not selectively bound to trophoblast or placental mesenchymal elements, their accounts of placental diaphorases are in direct conflict.

We prefer Hart's account of placental diaphorases (the work has been rechecked repeatedly in this laboratory in many specimens), which would explain his observation that NADP-dependent 17β-hydroxysteroid dehydrogenase is restricted to the trophoblast (Hart, 1966a). Our interpretation of placental 17β-hydroxysteroid dehydrogenase activity rests entirely on Hart's findings, which are illustrated in Fig. 87.

Trophoblastic 17β-hydroxysteroid dehydrogenase is NAD- or NADP-mediated and histochemically is highly specific for oestradiol. It may therefore be concerned in oestrogen metabolism or subserve a transhydrogenase function. By contrast, the 17β-hydroxysteroid dehydrogenase located in foetal mesenchyme and blood vessels is apparently NAD-linked and is apparently uninfluenced by A-ring configuration. It must be emphasized that this enzyme's apparent dependence on NAD may be secondary to a lack of NADP diaphorase, but its substrate-specificity is so different from that found in the trophoblast that it would seem reasonable to conclude that there are at least two placental 17β-hydroxysteroid dehydrogenases.

In summary, the trophoblastic 17β-hydroxysteroid dehydrogenase may rightly be termed oestradiol-17β-hydroxysteroid dehydrogenase, and it

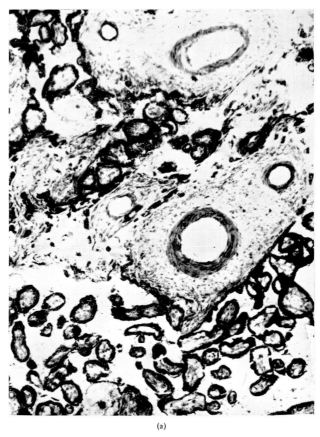

(a)

FIG. 87. (a) NAD-linked oestradiol-17β-dehydrogenase activity in trophoblast, vessels and perivascular stroma of term human placenta. × 100.

appears to be related in some way to steroid biosynthesis. The 17β-hydroxy-steroid dehydrogenase found in foetal mesenchyme and blood vessels is probably a distinct enzyme, and it is tempting to speculate that it may serve some barrier function in preventing biologically active 17β-hydroxysteroids from reaching the foetus by converting them to less active 17-keto forms.

Botte *et al.* (1966) described 17β-hydroxysteroid dehydrogenase in the trophoblastic giant cells and yolk-sac endodermal cells of the rat placenta, using oestradiol-17β and testosterone as substrates and both NAD and NADP as pyridine nucleotide co-factors. Oestriol and testosterone propionate were not suitable substrates. The presence of 17β-hydroxysteroid dehydro-genase activity and the 3β-hydroxysteroid dehydrogenase activity reported by Deane *et al.* (1962) and Botte *et al.* (1966) supports the biochemical evidence for placental secretion of progestogens and probable secretion of oestrogens put forward by Munemitsu and Segal (1959) as a result of experiments with parabiotic rats.

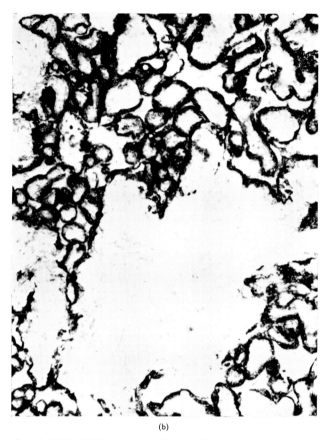

(b)

FIG. 87. Continued. (b) NADP-linked oestradiol-17β-dehydrogenase activity in an adjacent section of the same placenta. Formazan deposition is seen only in the trophoblast. × 100.

J. 20α- AND 20β-HYDROXYSTEROID DEHYDROGENASES

20α- and 20β-Hydroxysteroid dehydrogenases are involved in the metabolisms of progestogens. Balogh (1964), describing the histochemical demonstration of NADP-dependent 20α-hydroxysteroid dehydrogenase in the rat corpus luteum, states that rat placenta in the last week of gestation does not show evidence of this enzyme, and Weist and Forbes (1964) found that 20α-hydroxyprogesterone failed to maintain pregnancy in oophorectomized mice.

It has not proved possible to demonstrate 20α-hydroxysteroid dehydrogenase activity in human placenta in this laboratory with 20α-hydroxyprogesterone as substrate; 20α-hydroxyprogesterone, however, has been found in human liquor amnii (Lambert and Pennington, 1964) and in the placenta and blood of ewes (Short and Moore, 1959), and 20α-hydroxysteroid dehydro-

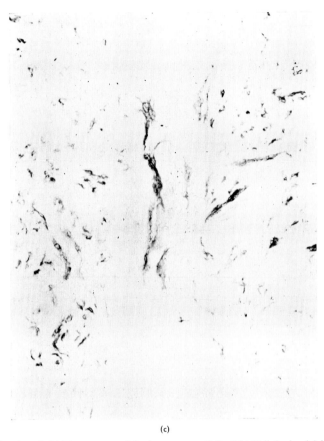

(c)

FIG. 87. Continued. (c) Testosterone dehydrogenase activity (NAD-linked only) is limited to the vessels and perivascular stroma. Term human placenta. × 100.

genase has been demonstrated biochemically in human placenta (Little *et al.*, 1959).

Lauritzen (1963) has shown that 20β-hydroxyprogesterone is a true progestogen in women, though only half as potent as progesterone itself with respect to its effects on uterus and vagina. Hart (1966a, b, c) failed to find convincing histochemical evidence of 20β-hydroxysteroid dehydrogenase in immature and term human placenta, in foetal membranes or in hydatidiform moles.

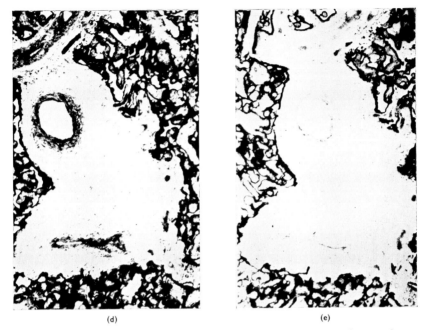

(d)   (e)

FIG. 87. Continued. (d) NAD-diaphorase is intense and ubiquitous. Term human placenta. ×60. (e) NADP diaphorase activity in an adjacent section. Even after 15 hours incubation very little activity is present in the mesenchyme, whereas strong activity is present in the trophoblast. ×60.

K. 21- AND 24-HYDROXYSTEROID DEHYDROGENASES

Baillie *et al.* (1966) failed to demonstrate 21- or 24-hydroxysteroid dehydrogenase activity in human placenta.

II. HYDATIDIFORM MOLES

Hydatidiform mole is characterized by trophoblastic proliferation, hydropic degeneration of the villous stroma and scantiness of blood vessels (Novak and Woodruff, 1962). There is more epithelial proliferation in that part of the mole which is attached to the uterine wall than in expelled vesicles, but the two layers of trophoblast are almost identical histologically with those in normal placenta.

Hart (1966c) examined hydatidiform moles histochemically for evidence of hydroxysteroid dehydrogenase activity and found that the range of activity closely resembled that of normal human placenta, both with regard to the range of hydroxysteroids utilized and the relative intensities of the reactions.

Strong 3β-, 16β- and oestradiol-17β-hydroxysteroid dehydrogenase activities (Fig. 88), NAD-linked, were invariably found in the trophoblast whenever the appropriate steroid substrates were employed. Weaker 3α- and poor 11β-hydroxysteroid dehydrogenase activities, NAD-linked, were present in five out of six moles examined for these enzymes, and poor 6β-hydroxysteroid dehydrogenase in only one out of six.

NADP-linked 3β, 16β- and oestradiol-17β-dehydrogenases were constantly present in the trophoblast; the intensity of reaction was variable but usually weak. Testosterone was not dehydrogenated; this is not surprising in view of the vascular distribution of placental testosterone 17β-dehydrogenase and the scantiness of blood vessels in hydatidiform moles. Warren and French (1965) demonstrated steroid sulphatase activity in hydatidiform moles, and the utilization of DHA sulphate as a substrate for 3β-hydroxysteroid dehydrogenase in moles (Hart, 1966c) accords with their report.

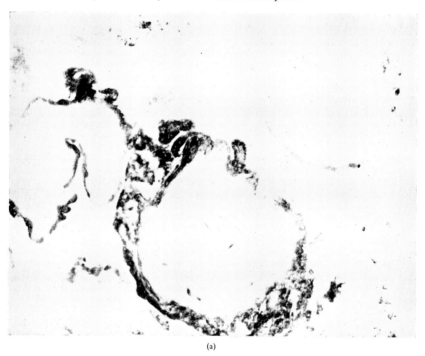

(a)

FIG. 88. (a) 3α-Hydroxysteroid dehydrogenase in the trophoblast of a hydatidiform mole. NAD-linked. × 100.

In the non-pregnant individual urinary oestriol is mainly derived from catabolism of oestrone and oestradiol; however, in normal pregnancy the majority of urinary oestriol is derived from sources other than maternal oestrone–oestradiol catabolism, although the mechanism of production is not clear. Patients with hydatidiform mole show an extremely small independent production of oestriol as compared with normal pregnant women (MacDonald and Siiteri, 1964); the relatively normal hydroxysteroid dehydrogenase

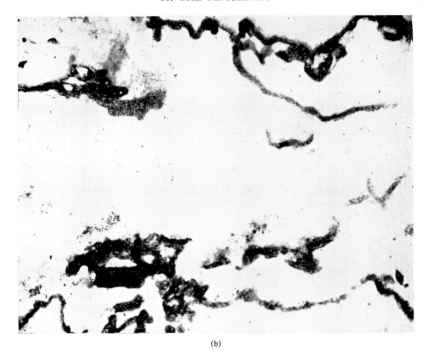

(b)

FIG. 88. Continued. (b) 3β-hydroxysteroid dehydrogenase activity. NAD-linked, in the trophoblast of a hydatidiform mole. × 150.

activity of mole trophoblast supports the suggestion that this lowered oestrogen production is secondary to inadequate access of maternal DHA sulphate due to the faulty development of foetal vasculature.

III. THE HUMAN FOETAL MEMBRANES

The extraplacental chorionic trophoblast layer was the most active, displaying 3α-, 3β-, 11β-, 16β- and 17β-oestradiol-hydroxysteroid dehydrogenase activities; the amniotic epithelium possessed weak 3α- and 3β-hydroxysteroid dehydrogenase and moderate 17β-hydroxysteroid dehydrogenase activities, and weak 3α- and 3β-hydroxysteroid dehydrogenases were present in connective tissue (Hart, 1966b). All activity demonstrated was NAD-linked (Fig. 89).

17β-Hydroxysteroid dehydrogenase activity was not seen when testosterone was employed as steroid substrate; in the term placenta, testosterone dehydrogenase activity is restricted to blood vessel walls (Hart, 1966a; Koide and Mitsudo, 1965). Since blood vessels are not present in the membranes, the absence of hydroxysteroid dehydrogenase activity with testosterone as substrate is confirmatory evidence of the vascular distribution of placental testosterone-17β-dehydrogenase.

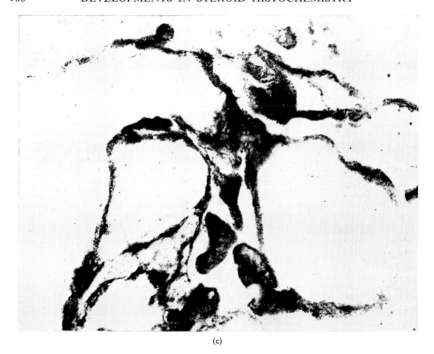

(c)

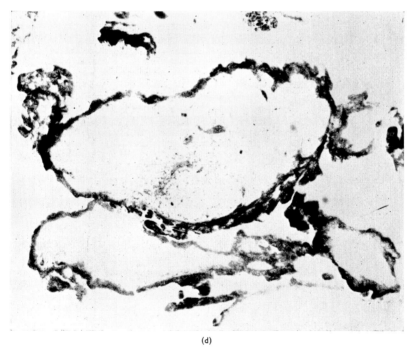

(d)

FIG. 88. Continued. (c) Intense 16β-hydroxysteroid dehydrogenase activity, NAD-linked, in an area of active trophoblastic proliferation in a hydatidiform mole. × 170. (d) NAD-linked oestradiol-17β-dehydrogenase activity in a hydatidiform mole. Comparison with part (a) (term placenta) draws attention to the scantiness of stroma and lack of blood vessels in hydatidiform mole. × 110.

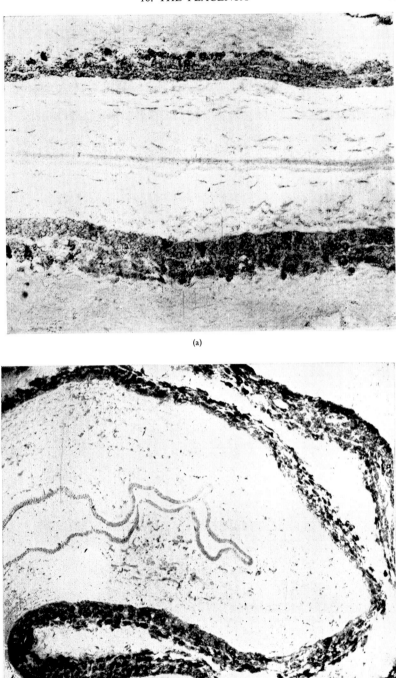

(a)

(b)

FIG. 89. (a) 3β-Hydroxysteroid dehydrogenase in term human foetal membranes. The reaction is strongest in the extra-placental trophoblast. × 180. (b) 16β-Hydroxysteroid dehydrogenase activity is intense in the trophoblast layer of the term human chorion. × 150.

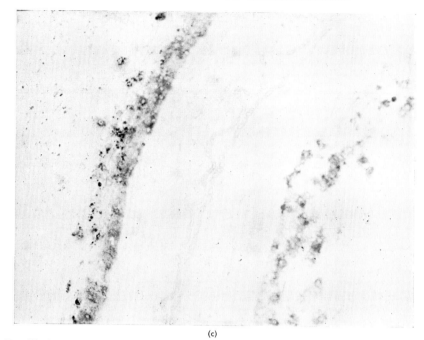

(c)

FIG. 89. Continued. (c) Oestradiol 17β-dehydrogenase in term human foetal membranes.
×220.

The foetal membranes have been shown to be metabolically active and the amnion can transport both fluid and electrolytes (Bourne and Lacy, 1960; Garby, 1957). Osinski (1960) found the human foetal membranes to be a rich source of 11β-hydroxysteroid dehydrogenase. The presence of a range of hydroxysteroid dehydrogenases indicates that the non-placental trophoblast is potentially capable of steroid hormone synthesis and metabolism.

A. THE YOLK-SAC

NAD and NADP diaphorases (Hart, 1966b) have been shown to occur in the mesenchymal and endodermal cells of the yolk-sac, a prerequisite for the histochemical demonstration of hydroxysteroid dehydrogenases. Oestradiol-17β-hydroxysteroid dehydrogenase activity is demonstrable with NAD and NADP in the endodermal (Fig. 90) and, to a lesser extent, in the mesenchymal cells of the rat (Botte *et al.*, 1966) and human yolk-sac (Hart, 1966b). 3α-, 3β-, 11β- and 16β-Hydroxysteroid dehydrogenases are, however, not histochemically demonstrable, and the hydroxysteroid dehydrogenase pattern in the yolk-sac is thus not one of steroid biosynthesis of the type established in the adrenal gland, gonads and placenta. The presence of a 17β-hydroxysteroid dehydrogenase in yolk-sac endoderm is of particular interest ontogenetically, in view of the existence of a 17β-hydroxysteroid dehydrogenase in comparable endodermal derivatives, including the duodenal mucosa (see Chapter 8) and liver (see Chapter 9).

Extra-regional and yolk-sac germ cells are known to occur in the human embryo (Fuss, 1911; Felix, 1912; Florian, 1931; Debeyre, 1933; Politzer, 1933), and Hart (1966b) confirmed their presence in the yolk-sac of a 14 mm embryo having endodermal 17β-hydroxysteroid dehydrogenase, using the peculiar presence in the germ cells of an alkaline phosphatase (McKay *et al.*, 1953).

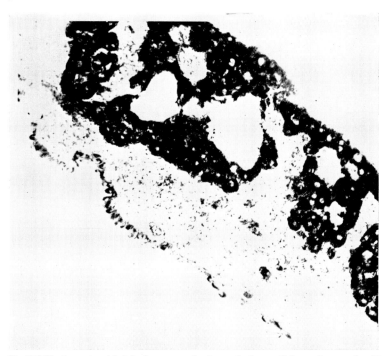

Fig. 90. 17β-Hydroxysteroid dehydrogenase in the endoderm of the yolk-sac of a 14 mm human foetus using oestradial as substrate. × 250.

REFERENCES

Adams, J. A., Jarabak, J. and Talalay, P. (1962). The steroid specificity of the 17β-hydroxysteroid dehydrogenase of human placenta. *J. Biol. Chem.* **237**, 3069–3073.

Axelrod, L. R. and Werthessen, N. T. (1961). Blood as a site for the conversion of the steroid hormones. *Endocrinology* **68**, 180–183.

Baillie, A. H., Ferguson, M. M. and Hart, D. McK. (1966b). Evidence of steroid metabolism and possible biosynthesis in the human genital ridge mesenchyme. *J. Clin. Endocrinol.* **26**, 738.

Baillie, A. H., Calman, K. C., Ferguson, M. M. and Hart, D. McK. (1966a). Histochemical utilisation of 3α-, 6β-, 11α-, 12α-, 16α-, 16β-, 17α-, 21- and 24-hydroxysteroids. *J. Endocrinol.* **34**, 1–12.

Baillie, A. H., Cameron, E. H. D., Griffiths, K. and Hart, D. McK. (1965a). 3β-Hydroxysteroid dehydrogenase in the adrenal gland and placenta. *J. Endocrinol.* **31**, 227–233.

Baillie, A. H., Ferguson, M. M., Calman, K. C. and Hart, D. McK. (1965b). Histochemical demonstration of 11β-hydroxysteroid dehydrogenase. *J. Endocrinol.* **33**, 119–125.

Baird, C. W. and Bush, I. E. (1960). Cortisol and cortisone content of amniotic fluid from diabetic and non-diabetic women. *Acta endocr. Copenh.* **34**, 97–104.

Balogh, K. (1964). A histochemical method for the demonstration of 20α-hydroxysteroid dehydrogenase activity in rat ovaries. *J. Histochem. Cytochem.* **12**, 670–673.

Baulieu, E. E. (1960). Three sulphate esters of 17-ketosteroids in the plasma of normal subjects and after administration of ACTH. *J. Clin. Endocrinol.* **20**, 900–904.

Baulieu, E. E. and Dray, F. (1963). Conversion of H^3-dehydroisoandrosterone (3β-hydroxy-Δ^5-androsten-17-one) sulfate to H^3-estrogens in normal pregnant women. *J. Clin. Endocrinol.* **23**, 1298–1301.

Bolté, E., Mancuso, S., Eriksson, G., Wiqvist, N. and Diczfalusy, E. (1964a). Studies on the aromatisation of neutral steroids in pregnant women. I. Aromatisation of C-19 steroids by placentas perfused in situ. *Acta Endocrinol.* **45**, 535–559.

Bolté, E., Mancuso, S., Eriksson, G., Wiqvist, N. and Diczfalusy, E. (1964b). Studies on the aromatisation of neutral steroids in pregnant women. II. Aromatisation of dehydroepiandrosterone and of its sulphate administered simultaneously into a uterine artery. *Acta Endocrinol.* **45**, 560–575.

Bolté, E., Mancuso, S., Eriksson, G., Wiqvist, N. and Diczfalusy, E. (1964c). Studies on the aromatisation of neutral steroids in pregnant women. III. Over-all aromatisation of dehydroepiandrosterone sulphate circulating in the foetal and maternal compartment. *Acta Endocrinol.* **45**, 576–599.

Botte, V., Materazzi, G. and Chieffi, G. (1966). Histochemical distribution of Δ^5-3β-hydroxysteroid dehydrogenase and 17α- and 17β-hydroxysteroid dehydrogenases in the placenta and foetal membranes of rat. *J. Endocrinol.* **34**, 179–183.

Bourne, G. L. and Lacy, D. (1960). Ultrastructure of human amnion and its possible relation to the circulation of amniotic fluid. *Nature* **186**, 952–954.

Breuer, H. and Knuppen, R. (1958). Metabolism of 16-oxo-oestrone by human liver slices *in vitro*. *Nature* **182**, 1512.

Breuer, H. and Nocke, L. (1959). Formation of oestriol-3, 16β, 17α by liver tissue *in vitro*. *Biochim. Biophys. Acta*. **36**, 271–272.

Deane, H. W., Rubin, B. L., Driks, E. C., Lobel, B. L. and Leipsner, G. (1962). Trophoblastic giant cells in placentas of rats and mice and their probable role in steroid-hormone production. *Endocrinology* **70**, 407–419.

Debeyre, A. (1933). Sur la présence de gonocytes chez un embryon humain au stade de la ligne primitive. *Compt. Rend. Assoc. Anat.* **28**, 240–250.

Felix, W. (1912). The development of the urogenital organs in: *Manual of Human Embryology* (Keibel and Mall), Vol. **2**, pp. 752–979 (Lippincott, Philadelphia).

Florian, J. (1931). "Urkeimzellen" bei einem 625μ langen menschlichen Embryo. *Anat. Anz.* **72**, 286.

Fuhrmann, K. (1961). Uber den histochemischen Nachweis der 3β-ol-Steroidde-hydrogenase-Activität in Geweben endokriner Organe. *Zentr. Gynackol.* **15**, 565–572.

Fuss, A. (1911). Ueber extraregionare Geschlechtszellen bei einem menschlichen Embryo von 4 Wochen. *Anat. Anz.* **39**, 407–409.

Garby, L. (1957). Studies on transfer of matter across membranes with special reference to the isolated human amniotic membrane and the exchange of amniotic fluid. *Acta Physiol. Scand. Suppl.* **40**, 137 (1957).

Goldberg, B., Jones, G. E. S. and Turner, D. A. (1963). Steroid 3β-ol dehydrogenase activity in human endocrine tissues. *Am. J. Obstet. Gynecol.* **86**, 349–359.

Hagerman, D. D. and Villee, C. A. (1959). Separation of human placental estrogen-sensitive transhydrogenase from estradiol-17β dehydrogenase. *J. Biol. Chem.* **234**, 2031–2036.

Hagerman, D. D., Villee, C. A. and Wellington, F. M. (1959). Separation of human placental estrogen-sensitive transhydrogenase from estradiol-17β dehydro-genase. *Federation Proc.* **18**, 240.

Hart, D. McK. (1966a). Hydroxysteroid dehydrogenase activity in normal, human placenta from 6 weeks to 42 weeks of gestation. *J. Endocrinol.* **35**, 255–262.

Hart, D. McK. (1966b). The histochemical distribution of hydroxysteroid dehydro-genases in the human foetal membranes at term. *Histochemie* **6**, 17–23.

Hart, D. McK. (1966c). Histochemical demonstration of hydroxysteroid dehydro-genases in hydatidiform moles. *Obstet. Gynecol.* **27**, 766–771.

Hart, D. McK. (1966d). Histochemical investigation of the localisation of placental 17β-hydroxysteroid dehydrogenases. M. D. Thesis. University of Glasgow.

Hart, D. McK. (1966e). Evidence of steroid metabolism in a human yolk sac. In: M.D. Thesis. University of Glasgow.

Iwata, K. (1959). *Tokyo Jikeikai Ika Daigaku Zasshi* **74**, 927 (quoted by Dorfman and Ungar, 1965, in *Metabolism of Steroid Hormones* (Academic Press, New York).

Jarabak, J., Adams, J. A., Williams-Ashman, H. G. and Talalay, P. (1962). Purifica-tion of a 17β-hydroxysteroid dehydrogenase of human placenta and studies on its transhydrogenase function. *J. Biol. Chem.* **237**, 345–357.

Kellogg, D. A. and Glenner, G. G. (1960). Histochemical localisation of human, term placental 17β-oestradiol dehydrogenases; implications for the trans-hydrogenase reaction. *Nature* **187**, 763–764.

Klausner, D. A. and Ryan, K. J. (1964). Estriol secretion by the human term placenta. *J. Clin. Endocrinol.* **24**, 101–104.

Kleiner, H., Wilkin, P. and Snoeck, J. (1962). *Geburtsh. Frauenheilk.* **22**, 986.

Koide, S. S. and Mitsudo, S. M. (1965). Histochemical study of 3β- and 17β-hydroxysteroid dehydrogenases in human term placenta. *Endocrinology* **76**, 403–407.

Lambert, M. and Pennington, G. W. (1964). Isolation and identification of the 20β-hydroxyderivatives of 6β-hydroxycortisol and 6β-hydroxycortisone in liquor amnii. *Nature* **203**, 656.

Langer, L. J., Alexander, J. A. and Engel, L. L. (1959). Human placental estradiol-17β-dehydrogenase. II. Kinetics and substrate specificities. *J. Biol. Chem.* **234**, 2,609–2,614.

Langer, L. J. and Engel, L. L. (1958). Human placental estradiol-17β-dehydro-genase. I. Concentration, characterisation and assay. *J. Biol. Chem.* **233**, 583–588.

Lauritzen, C. (1963). Biologische Wirkungen des 20β-Hydroxypregn-4-en-3-on. *Acta Endocrinol.* **44**, 225–236.

Levitz, M., Condon, G. P. and Dancis, J. (1956). The interconversion of estrone and estradiol in the perfused human placenta. *Endocrinology* **58**, 376–380.

Levitz, M., Rosen, M. F. and Twombly, G. H. (1960). Interconversions of 16-oxygenated estrogens. II. Metabolism of 16-keto estradiol 17β 16-C^{14} in man. *Arch. Biochim. Biophys.* **88**, 212–215.

Levitz, M., Spitzer, T. R. and Twombly, G. H. (1958). Interconversions of 16-oxygenated estrogens. I. The synthesis of estriol 16-C^{14} and its metabolism in man. *J. Biol. Chem.* **231**, 787–797.

Little, B., Dimartinis, J. and Nyholm, B. (1959). The conversion of progesterone to Δ^4-pregnene-20α-ol, 3-one by human placenta *in vitro*. *Acta Endocrinol.* **30**, 530–538.

Lobel, B. L., Deane, H. W. and Romney, S. L. (1962). Enzymic histochemistry of the villous portion of the human placenta from six weeks of gestation to term. *Am. J. Obstet. Gynecol.* **83**, 295–299.

MacDonald, P. C. and Siiteri, P. K. (1964). Study of estrogen production in women with hydatidiform mole. *J. Clin. Endocrinol.* **24**, 685–690.

McKay, D. G., Hertig, A. T., Adams, E. C. and Danzinger, S. (1953). Histochemical observations on the germ cells of human embryos. *Anat. Record* **117**, 201–219.

Munemitsu, S. and Segal, S. J. (1959). Endocrine role of rat placenta as revealed by experiments in parabiosis. *Arch. Anat. Microscop. Morphol. Exptl.* **48**, 173–188.

Novak, E. R. and Woodruff, J. D. (1962). *Obstetric and Gynecologic Pathology* 5th edn. (Saunders, Philadelphia).

Osinski, P. A. (1960). Steroid 11β-ol dehydrogenase in human placenta. *Nature* **187**, 777.

Politzer, T. (1933). Die Keimbahn des Menschen. Zeit. Ges. Anat. abt. I. *Z. Anat. Entwicklungsgeschichte* **100**, 331–361.

Pulkkinen, M. O. (1961). Arylsulphatase and the hydrolysis of some steroid sulphates in developing organism and placenta. Acta Physiol. Scand. *Suppl.* **52**, 7–92.

Ryan, K. J. (1960). Metabolism of 16-keto-estrone by human placenta. *Endocrinology* **66**, 491–494.

Ryan, K. J. and Engel, L. L. (1953). The interconversion of estrone and estradiol by human tissue slices. *Endocrinology* **52**, 287–291.

Schiebler, T. H. and Knoop, A. (1959). Histochemische und Elektronen-mikroskopische untersuchungen an der rattenplazenta. *Z. Zellforsch.* **50**, 494–552.

Short, R. V. and Moore, N. W. (1959). Progesterone in blood. V. Progesterone and 20α-hydroxypregn-4-en-3-one in the placenta and blood of ewes. *J. Endocrinol.* **19**, 288–293.

Siiteri, P. K. and MacDonald, P. C. (1963). The utilisation of circulating dehydroepiandrosterone sulphate for oestrogen synthesis during human pregnancy. *Steroids* **2**, 713–730.

Talalay, P., Hurlock, B. and Williams-Ashman, H G. (1958a). On a co-enzymatic function of estradiol-17β. *Proc. Natl. Acad. Sc . U.S.* **44**, 862–884.

Talalay, P. and Williams-Ashman, H. G. (1958b). Activation of hydrogen transfer between pyridine nucleotides by steroid hormones. *Proc. Natl. Acad. Sci. U.S.* **44**, 15–26.

Troen, P. (1961). Perfusion studies of the human placenta. II. Metabolism of C^{14}-17β-estradiol with and without added human chorionic gonadotropin. *J. Clin. Endocrinol.* **21**, 895–908.

Troen, P. (1962). Excerpta Med. Intern. Congr. Ser. **51**, 269. Quoted in: *Metabolism of Steroid Hormones* (Dorfman and Ungar) (Academic Press, New York, 1965).

Villee, C. A. (1961). Die Beeinflussung von Enzymen in Uterus und Placenta durch Oestrogene. *Klin. Wochschr.* **39**, 173–178.

Warren, J. C. and French, A. P. (1965). Distribution of steroid sulfatase in human tissues. *J. Clin. Endocrinol.* **25**, 278–285.

Warren, J. C. and Timberlake, C. E. (1962). Steroid sulfatase in the human placenta. *J. Clin. Endocrin.* **22**, 1148–1151.

Wattenberg, L. W. (1958). Microscopic histochemical demonstration of steroid-3β-ol dehydrogenase in tissue sections. *J. Histochem. Cytochem.* **6**, 225–232.

Weist, W. G. and Forbes, T. R. (1964). Failure of 20α-Hydroxy-Δ^4-pregnen-3-one and 20β-hydroxy-Δ^4-pregnen-3-one to maintain pregnancy in ovariectomised mice. *Endocrinology* **74**, 149–150.

Wislocki, G. B. and Dempsey, E. W. (1955). Electron microscopy of the placenta of the rat. *Anat. Record* **123**, 33–63.

CHAPTER 11

Experimental Modifications

I. THE ADRENAL GLANDS

Hypophysectomy is known to lead to progressive atrophy of the inner two zones of the adrenal cortex in ordinary histological preparations, the residual cells becoming markedly eosinophilic. Only the glomerular zone has been shown to be secretory after hypophysectomy (Rauschkolb et al., 1956) and it remains histologically normal. Samuels and Helmreich (1956) noted a fall in 3β-hydroxysteroid dehydrogenase activity in the homogenated adrenal glands of hypophysectomized rats; this reduction in 3β-hydroxysteroid dehydrogenase is progressive and related to the steady atrophy of the gland, but the activity per unit mass does not drop significantly biochemically. Histochemically (Levy et al., 1959; Fuhrmann, 1963) 3β- and 17β-hydroxysteroid dehydrogenase activity has been shown not to change in rat or rabbit adrenal glands during the first few days after hypophysectomy, both enzymes being found throughout the fascicular and reticular zones in these animals; thereafter activity gradually declines, and by the fiftieth day after hypophysectomy the inner half of the cortex is almost inactive.

ACTH administration (Levy et al., 1959; Fuhrmann, 1963) effectively prevents or reverses the reduction in adrenal 3β-hydroxysteroid dehydrogenase activity in hypophysectomized animals. In intact mice (Pearson et al., 1964), ACTH administration causes a transient increase in 3β-hydroxysteroid dehydrogenase activity in the adrenal gland. ACTH is known to stimulate adrenal phosphorylase, and this has led to the hypothesis that the existing levels of cyclic AMP are influenced by ACTH, which mechanism in turn controls the availability of reduced NADP for steroid metabolism (Hall and Eik-Nes, 1962). The histochemical results indicate a selective loss of active 3β-hydroxysteroid dehydrogenase in the adrenal glands of hypophysectomized animals after a period of time. This loss could be explained by diminished protein synthesis but further work is required on this subject.

Marx and Deane (1963) have shown that severe salt depletion produced by a low-sodium diet results in a tenfold hypertrophy of the zona glomerulosa in rats over several weeks, together with a steady rise in its contained 3β-hydroxysteroid dehydrogenase. Similar changes follow the administration of angio-tension (Marx et al., 1963) in rats, and the degree of glomerular hypertrophy is proportional to the dosage and duration of administration, as is the level of glomerular 3β-hydroxysteroid dehydrogenase.

According to Pearson et al. (1964), cold stress in mice leads to a 50% reduction in 3β-hydroxysteroid dehydrogenase activity in the zona glomerulosa, whereas only a slight drop occurs in the activity of the enzyme in the fascicular and reticular zones. Surgical trauma produces an initial (18 hours) fall in mouse adrenal 3β-hydroxysteroid dehydrogenase, followed by a substantial increase in activity. Pearson et al. (1964) also describe progressive reduction in adrenal 3β-hydroxysteroid dehydrogenase in mice with spontaneous mammary carcinoma, but the significance of this observation is unclear.

Freses et al. (1965) record a somewhat unexpected reduction in Δ^5-3β-hydroxysteroid dehydrogenase activity in rat adrenal glands after ACTH administration. Further work is needed to resolve the various conflicting opinions in this experimental field.

II. THE TESTIS

The ability of gonadotrophins to raise the testicular production of testosterone and other steroids is well known in man (Landau and Laves, 1959; Korenman et al., 1963; Dupre et al., 1964) and various animals, and attention has recently been turning to the possible site of action of ICSH. Hall (1963) noted that ICSH increases the production of testosterone from [1-^{14}C]acetate by rabbit testis slices and considered that ICSH stimulates the biosynthetic pathway between acetate and testosterone at some point(s) after cholesterol. As a result of further studies, Hall and Eik-Nes (1964) concluded that, in the rabbit at least, gonadotrophic stimulation of testicular steroidogenesis was principally effected between cholesterol and pregnenolone.

Biochemically (Samuels and Helmreich, 1956), testicular 3β-hydroxysteroid dehydrogenase activity rises immediately after hypophysectomy, owing to gonadotrophin release from the pituitary at operation. The total activity per testis drops rapidly, after the initial transient rise, for five or six days and then more slowly for another sixty days or so. Chorionic gonadotrophin reverses the results of hypophysectomy if administered to the experimental animal, but is without effect if added to homogenates of atrophic testes from hypophysectomized animals.

Niemi and Ikonen (1962) noted that histochemically demonstrable Δ^5-3β-hydroxysteroid dehydrogenase in the interstitium of rat testes falls markedly after hypophysectomy, while chorionic gonadotrophin administration greatly increases Leydig cell 3β-hydroxysteroid dehydrogenase. In addition, we have noted that hypophysectomy in rats leads to some reduction in 3α-, 11β-, 16β- and 17β-hydroxysteroid dehydrogenases in the Leydig cells, but abolition of activity is far from complete six weeks after operation. A similar reduction in enzyme activity occurs in the testes of hamsters exposed to severe cold ($-6°$) for up to four weeks. Accompanying the progressive fall in dehydrogenase activity, testicular weight drops to 10% of control levels. Administration of testosterone propionate reduces 3β-hydroxysteroid dehydrogenase in the rat Leydig cells (Niemi and Ikonen, 1962), and oestrogen therapy for prostatic carcinoma in man (Baillie and Mack, 1966) wipes out testicular 3α-, 3β-, 11β-

16β-, 17β- and 20β-hydroxysteroid dehydrogenases as histochemically demonstrable enzymes.

Arvy (1962), Chieffi and Botte (1963) and Cavallero *et al.* (1963) have shown that administration of FSH, LH or chorionic gonadotrophin leads to an increase in the histochemical activity of Δ^5-3β-hydroxysteroid dehydrogenase in the Leydig cells. The biochemical and histochemical observations can be fully explained by assuming that pituitary or placental ICSH controls the rate of synthesis of hydroxysteroid dehydrogenases, either from amino acids or from a more complex but inactive precursor, and evidence has been adduced (Samuels and Helmreich, 1956; Hall and Eik-Nes, 1964) to show that ICSH directly stimulates testicular protein synthesis from [1-^{14}C] tryptophan and [1-^{14}C]valine both *in vivo* and *in vitro*. Oestrogens, and to a lesser extent testosterone, presumably act by depressing pituitary production of ICSH, but a local effect on the Leydig cells cannot yet be fully excluded.

Food deprivation (Niemi and Ikonen, 1962) sufficient to cause a 50% fall in body weight reduces but does not eliminate rat testicular 3β-hydroxysteroid dehydrogenase. Partial ischaemia (Baillie and Mack, 1966) has little effect on histochemically demonstrable hydroxysteroid dehydrogenases in the human testis; total ischaemia, on the other hand, leads to infarction and complete loss of hydroxysteroid dehydrogenase activity, as one would expect.

Favino *et al.* (1966) noted that cadmium-poisoned testes retain islets of histochemically normal Leydig cells, just deep to the tunica albuginea testis. These cells exhibit 3β-, 11β-, 16β- and 17β-hydroxysteroid dehydrogenases and are sufficient to account for the continuing, but much reduced, testicular production of testosterone and androstenedione. The necrotic interior of the cadmium-poisoned testis is invaded by atypical mesenchymal cells from the tunica albuginea which exhibit weak 3α- and 16β-hydroxysteroid dehydrogenase activity. The significance of the latter cells is unclear.

III. THE OVARY

Hypophysectomy in the female ends follicular maturation and leads to regression of the interstitial tissue. At the same time, 3β-hydroxysteroid dehydrogenase shows a progressive decline in the interstitial tissue (Levy *et al.*, 1959), and three months after operation no 3β-hydroxysteroid dehydrogenase is demonstrable (Taylor, 1961). The response of the corpora lutea differed in these two experiments: Levy *et al.* (1959) found no decline in 3β-hydroxy-steroid dehydrogenase content of the corpora lutea eleven weeks after hypophysectomy, whereas Taylor (1961) failed to detect 3β-hydroxysteroid dehydrogenase in corpora lutea three months after operation.

Human chorionic gonadotrophin (Taylor, 1961) restores 3β-hydroxysteroid dehydrogenase activity in rat ovarian tissues after hypophysectomy. In intact immature rats (Rubin and Deane, 1965) gonadotrophins were administered in a manner designed to produce superovulation, and, in the very young animals, a marked increase in 3β-hydroxysteroid dehydrogenase activity followed. As the intact animals aged they responded less well to parenteral gonadotrophins. In mature animals responses were poorer and less predictable; the luteal tissue increased in volume but its 3β-hydroxysteroid dehydrogenase content appeared to remain constant. Similar results are recorded by Botte and Del Bianco (1962).

Following hemicastration (Rubin *et al.*, 1965), the weight of the remaining ovary increases regularly; Δ^5-3β-hydroxysteroid dehydrogenase activity as a rule also increases, but the two changes are not always parallel. The bulk of the conclusions in the paper, however, rest on biochemical rather than histochemical data.

Goldman *et al.* (1965) have investigated the effects of a synthetic steroidal inhibitor, 2α-cyano-4,4,17α-trimethyl-androst-5-on-17β-ol-3-one, on the steroid-producing tissues of the rat. The ovarian and placental results form an interesting contrast in that ovarian Δ^5-3β-hydroxysteroid dehydrogenase is reduced while the corpora lutea undergo hyperplasia, but placental 17β-hydroxysteroid dehydrogenase activity seems to be unaffected.

REFERENCES

Arvy, L. (1962). Action de l'hormone gonadotrope choriale sur quelques activités enzymatiques testiculaires chez le Rat. *Compt. Rend.* **255**, 1532–1534.

Baillie, A. H. and Mack, W. S. (1966). Hydroxysteroid dehydrogenases in normal and abnormal human testes. *J. Endocrinol.* **35**, 239–248.

Botte, V. and Del Bianco, C. (1962). Studies of the histological modifications and of the changes of the histochemical distribution of lipids and steroid-3β-ol dehydrogenase in the ovaries of immature rats treated with gonadotrophins. *Arch. Ostet. Ginecol.* **67**, 653–665.

Cavallero, C., Martinazzi, M., Baroni, C. and Magrini, U. (1963). Pituitary control of mouse testis in hereditary dwarfism; Histological and cytochemical observations. *Gen. Comp. Endocrinol.* **3**, 636–643.

Chieffi, G. and Botte, V. (1963). *Riv. Istoch. Norm. Patol.* **9**, 172–174.

Dupre, J., Brooks, R. V., Hyde, R., London, D. R., Prunty, F. T. G. and Self, J. B. (1964). Preliminary observations on testosterone in testicular vein blood from abnormal human testes. *J. Endocrinol.* **29**, VII.

Favino, A., Baillie, A. H. and Griffiths, K. (1966). Androgen synthesis by the testes and adrenal glands of cadmium chloride poisoned rats. *J. Endocrinol.* (in press).

Freses, A. T., Diaz, J. and Falen, J. (1965). Efecto de ACTH, dexametusona y progesterona sobre la actividad de 3β-ol-esteroide deshidrogenasa de la suprarrenal de rata albina. Estudio histoquimico. *Rev. Iber. Endocrinol.* **12**, 5–14.

Fuhrmann, K. (1963). Histochemische Untersuchungen uber Hydroxysteroid dehydrogenase-aktivitat in nebennieren und eierstocken von ratten und kaninchen. *Arch. Gynaekol.* **197**, 583–600.

Goldman, A. S., Yakovac, W. C. and Bongiovanni, A. M. (1965). Persistent effects of a synthetic androstene derivative on activities of 3β-hydroxysteroid dehydrogenase and glucose-6-phosphate dehydrogenase in rats. *Endocrinology* **77**, 1105–1118.

Hall, P. F. (1963). The effect of interstitial-cell-stimulating hormone on the bio-synthesis of testicular cholesterol from acetate-1-C^{14}. *Biochemistry* **2**, 1232–1237.

Hall, P. F. and Eik-Nes, K. B. (1962). The action of gonadotropic hormones upon rabbit testis *in vitro. Biochim. Biophys. Acta* **63**, 411–422.

Hall, P. F. and Eik-Nes, K. B. (1964). The effect of interstitial cell-stimulating hormone on the production of pregnenolone by rabbit testis in the presence of an inhibitor of 17α-hydroxylase. *Biochim. Biophys. Acta* **86**, 604–609.

Korenman, S. G., Wilson, H. and Lipsett, M. B. (1963). Testosterone production rates in normal adults. *J. Clin. Invest.* **42**, 1753–1760.

Landau, R. L. and Laves, M. L. (1959). Urinary pregnanetriol of testicular origin. *J. Clin. Endocrinol.* **19**, 1344–1404.

Levy, H., Deane, H. W. and Rubin, B. L. (1959). Visualization of steroid-3β-ol-dehydrogenase activity in tissues of intact and hypophysectomised rats. *Endocrinology* **65**, 932–943.

Marx, A. J. and Deane, H. W. (1963). Histophysiologic changes in the kidney and adrenal cortex in rats on a low sodium diet. *Endocrinology* **73**, 317–328.

Marx, A. J., Deane, H. W., Mowles, T. F. and Sheppard, H. (1963). Chronic administration of angiotensin in rats: changes in blood pressure, renal and adrenal histophysiology and aldosterone production. *Endocrinology* **73**, 329–337.

Niemi, M. and Ikonen, M. (1962). Cytochemistry of oxidative enzyme systems in the Leydig cells of the rat testis and their functional significance. *Endocrinology* **70**, 167–174.

Pearson, B., Wolf, P., Grose, F. and Andrews, M. (1964). The histochemistry of 3β-hydroxysteroid dehydrogenase. I. With special reference to adrenal glands, as affected by ACTH, cold, trauma and tumor. *Am. J. Clin. Pathol.* **41**, 256–265.

Rauschkolb, E. W., Farrell, G. L. and Koletzky, S. (1956). Aldosterone secretion after hypophysectomy. *Am. J. Physiol.* **184**, 55.

Rubin, B. L. and Deane, H. W. (1965). Effects of superovulation on ovarian Δ^5-3β-hydroxysteroid dehydrogenase activity in rats of different ages. *Endocrinology* **76**, 382–389.

Rubin, B. L., Hamilton, J. A., Karlson, T. J. and Tufaro, R. I. (1965). Effect of the age of the rat at the time of hemicastration on the weight estimated secretory activity and Δ^5-3β-hydroxysteroid dehydrogenase activity of the remaining ovary. *Endocrinology* **77**, 909–916.

Samuels, L. T. and Helmreich, M. L. (1956). The influence of chorionic gonadotropin on the 3β-ol dehydrogenase activity of testes and adrenals. *Endocrinology* **58**, 435–442.

Taylor, F. B. (1961). Histochemical changes in the ovaries of normal and experi-mentally treated rats. *Acta Endocrinol.* **36**, 361–374.

Author Index

Numbers in italics are the pages on which the references are listed

A

Aakvaag, A., 41, *67*
Acevedo, H. F., 56, *67*
Acosta, A., 75, 96, *97*
Adams, E. C., 35, *38*, 169, *172*
Adams, J. A., 15, 21, *22*, *24*, 158, *169*, *171*
Alexander, F., 81, *100*
Alexander, J. A., 15, *24*, 158, *172*
Allen, E., 95, *102*
Allen, W. M., 81, *100*
Alonso, C., 74, *98*
Anderson, D., 37, *38*, 59, *70*
Andrada, J. A., 46, *70*
Andrews, M., 104, *119*, 174, 175, *178*
Aoshima, Y., 129, 131, *132*, 146, 147, *149*
Arnold, J., 103, *116*
Arvy, L., 45, *67*, 104, *116*, 176, *177*
Axelrod, L. R., 56, *67*, 152, *169*
Ayres, P. J., 114, *116*

B

Baggett, B., 51, 52, 61, *71*, 147, *150*
Baillie, A. H., 2, 6, 13, *22*, *23*, *24*, 27, 28, 29, 31, *33*, 35, 37, *37*, *38*, 39, 40, 42, 43, 44, 45, 46, 47, 48, 49, 50, 52, 53, 54, 55, 56, 58, 59, 62, *67*, *69*, 73, 74, 76, 78, 80, 82, 83, 84, 85, 87, 88, 90, 91, 96, *97*, *99*, *102*, 103, 104, 105, 107, 108, 109, 110, 111, 112, 114, *116*, *118*, 120, 121, 125, 126, 127, 130, *132*, 134, 135, 136, 139, 140, *140*, 143, 144, 145, 146, *149*, 152, 155, 156, 157, 158, 163, *169*, *170*, 175, 176, *177*
Baird, C. W., 156, *170*
Balestreri, R., 147, *149*
Balogh, K., 2, 8, 21, *23*, 88, *97*, 148, *149*, 161, *170*
Bandi, L., 105, *119*

Bara, G., 76, *97*
Baron, D. N., 80, *97*, 129, 130, *132*
Baroni, C., 45, *68*, 176, *177*
Bassett, D. L., 72, *98*
Baulieu, E. E., 106, *116*, 153, 154, *170*
Bell, G. H., 135, *141*
Bell, L. G. E., 4, *23*
Bellamy, D., 114, *119*
Benard, H., 145, *149*
Berthrong, M., 59, *67*
Beyer, K. F., 11, *23*, 41, *67*
Birchall, K., 130, *132*
Bitensky, L., 3, 4, 8, *23*
Björkman, N., 89, *97*
Bloch, B., 104, *116*
Bloch, E., 81, *97*
Bloch, K., 16, *23*
Bloom, W., 134, *141*
Bolté, E., 106, *119*, 154, *170*
Bompiani, A., 108, *118*
Bongiovanni, A. M., 45, 46, 54, *69*, 73, 77, 78, 80, *99*, 104, 105, *117*, *118*, 127, *132*, 136, *141*, 146, *150*, 177, *177*
Borkowf, H. I., 40, 45, 46, 54, 55, *68*, 73, 76, 79, 81, 86, 87, *99*
Botte, V., 45, *67*, *68*, *71*, 75, 76, 90, *97*, *98*, 154, 155, 160, 161, 168, *171*, 176, *177*
Bourne, G. L., 168, *170*
Bowerman, A. M., 89, *97*
Bradbury, S., 9, *23*
Brambell, F. W. R., 37, *37*, 91, *97*
Breuer, H., 20, *23*, 50, 52, 54, 61, *67*, *68*, *71*, 83, 86, 88, *97*, *100*, 147, *149*, 156, 157, *170*
Brinck-Johnsen, T., 41, *67*
Brooks, R. V., 175, *177*
Bulbrook, R. D., 114, *117*
Bullough, W. S., 95, *97*
Burley, J., 50, *71*
Bush, I. E., 156, *170*

179